W0050037

Imaging of Ulcerative Colitis

Massimo Tonolini

Editor

Imaging of Ulcerative Colitis

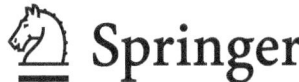 Springer

Editor
Massimo Tonolini
Radiology Department
Luigi Sacco University Hospital
Milan
Italy

ISBN 978-88-470-5408-0   ISBN 978-88-470-5409-7   (eBook)
DOI 10.1007/978-88-470-5409-7
Springer Milan Heidelberg New York Dordrecht London

Library of Congress Control Number: 2013951123

Printed on acid-free paper

Springer is part of Springer Science+Business Media (www.springer.com)

To Rita
We share everything

Preface

For the past 8 years I have been working at the "Luigi Sacco" Hospital in Milan, which mainly specializes in the care of infectious diseases and HIV and has become one of the leading centres for the treatment of chronic inflammatory bowel diseases.

In 2012, Professor Giovanni Maconi and I devised and edited a book about perianal inflammatory diseases, which encompassed the clinical, surgical, and radiological experience gained at our hospital, particularly in patients with Crohn's disease. Shortly after its publication by Springer, I asked the same team (including specialists in gastroenterology, surgery, and diagnostic imaging) to cooperate once more in order to produce this volume dealing with state-of-the-art cross-sectional imaging of ulcerative colitis.

The idea for this new book originates from the steadily increasing role of diagnostic imaging in the care of patients with chronic inflammatory bowel diseases. Fifteen years ago, during my residency at the San Paolo Hospital, I was trained in conventional gastrointestinal radiology. At that time, radiologists encountered few patients with ulcerative colitis, and usually when barium enema was requested. Meticulous double-contrast technique allowed demonstration of the subtle mucosal changes characteristic of the disease, and of advanced stages with shortened, nondistensible colon with loss of haustral folds were easily depicted.

Many years have passed, during which dramatic advancements have occurred in the medical and surgical treatment of patients with chronic inflammatory bowel diseases and in diagnostic imaging of intestinal disorders with ultrasound, multidetector CT, and MRI. As a result, there has been a progressive increase in the role of radiological modalities and their potential for complementing (and sometimes obviating) endoscopy in both urgent and elective conditions. Cross-sectional imaging is currently essential to comprehensively assess the colonic disease distribution and severity, its extraintestinal complications and multisystemic manifestations.

Therefore, the rationale for this book is to provide gastroenterologists, surgeons, and radiologists involved in the care of patients with ulcerative colitis with an increased familiarity with the role of diagnostic techniques in acute and elective conditions, and with the cross-sectional imaging appearances of ulcerative colitis, its mimics, and associated extraintestinal manifestations. Furthermore, since ileal pouch surgery is increasingly and successfully performed, knowledge of normal and abnormal postoperative appearances is needed in order to correctly perform and interpret imaging studies in operated patients.

As the editor of this volume, I would like to thank all my colleagues who have contributed to its production. We all hope it will be helpful to other radiologists and clinicians faced with different situations in the care of patients with chronic inflammatory bowel diseases.

Milan, October 2013   Massimo Tonolini

Contents

Introduction

Massimo Tonolini

As defined by the current guidelines of the European Crohn's and Colitis Organization (ECCO), which have been recently revised in 2012, Ulcerative Colitis (UC) is a life-long disease whose precise aetiology is unknown, that probably arises from an interaction between genetic and environmental factors. Pathologically, UC is a chronic inflammatory condition involving a non-granulomatous mucosal inflammation that starts from the rectum and extends proximally in a continuous, confluent manner to affect a variable extent of the colon or its entire mucosal surface [1, 2].

Nowadays, UC is observed predominantly in the developed world, and its incidence is reportedly increasing in Southern and developing countries. Characterized by a relapsing and remitting course, UC affects both sexes equally and usually presents in late adolescence and early adulthood. A second, smaller peak of incidence is observed after the fifth decade of life. The onset of UC is often insidious. Symptoms generally reflect the severity and extent of the disease, and most commonly include bloody diarrhoea, rectal bleeding and/or urgency [1, 2].

The diagnosis of UC is established upon a combination of medical history, clinical evaluation, and consistent endoscopic and histological findings. Traditionally, diagnostic imaging of UC relied on double-contrast barium enema, a modality which in experienced hands could provide useful information concerning the extent of colonic disease, although limited to the mucosal surface. The characteristic radiographic appearances include a continuous disease with invariable rectal involvement, a diffuse granularity or stippled pattern of the mucosa, pseudopolyps in a denuded flat mucosal surface, and a shortened, rigid and narrow colon with loss of normal haustral folds in advanced stages [1, 3, 4].

In recent years, diagnostic imaging modalities such as multidetector computed tomography (MDCT), magnetic resonance imaging (MRI) and ultrasound have undergone dramatic technical improvements, and are increasingly employed at referral centres to investigate UC patients in both urgent and elective settings. Complementary to endoscopy, cross-sectional imaging can assess the thickness and structure of the intestinal wall, as well as associated abnormalities of the perivisceral fat planes and surrounding organs. Therefore, imaging studies are optimally suited to comprehensively investigate the intestinal disease, associated perivisceral changes and extraintestinal manifestations [5–7].

For instance, since the intestinal extent of UC influences prognosis and dictates patient management and surveillance, the disease distribution classified according to the Montreal criteria may be investigated by means of water enema MDCT colonography or MRI in selected cases, such as proximally to an impassable stricture [1, 2].

M. Tonolini (✉)
Radiology Department, "Luigi Sacco" University Hospital, Via G.B. Grassi 74, 20157 Milan, Italy
e-mail: mtonolini@sirm.org

M. Tonolini (ed.), *Imaging of Ulcerative Colitis*,
DOI: 10.1007/978-88-470-5409-7_1, © Springer-Verlag Italia 2014

A potentially life-threatening condition, acute severe UC occurs in 15 % of patients, includes systemic symptoms such as malaise, vomiting, abdominal pain and fever, and represents an indication for in-hospital treatment. Although plain radiographs retain their traditional value in the initial assessment of patients with suspected severe UC, MDCT and MRI are increasingly employed to provide an earlier diagnosis, differentiate from other causes of acute abdomen, identify possible complications such as perforation or abscess collections, obviate the risk for endoscopy in a critical situation, allow intensive medical treatment and provide support for timely surgery [8, 9].

Furthermore, cross-sectional imaging is necessary to assess associated extraintestinal manifestations of UC that require a specific treatment approach, such as primary sclerosing cholangitis, portal venous system thrombosis and arthritis [10–16].

Patients with UC notoriously have an increased risk of developing colorectal cancer (CRC) compared to the general population, which is reported in the range 2.1–7.5 % and varies according to the extent of UC, the disease duration and to other factors such as associated sclerosing cholangitis, persistent inflammation and positive family history of CRC. Periodic surveillance colonoscopy is performed with the aim to reduce CRC-related morbidity and mortality, and identify those patients with high grade dysplasia and cancer that require proctocolectomy. Cross-sectional imaging can detect and stage neoplastic abnormalities such as CRC and anal carcinoma [17, 18].

Although with limited incidence compared to Crohn's disease, patients with UC may suffer from perianal inflammatory changes including fistulas and abscesses, sometimes involving the genital tract. These complications benefit from focused ultrasound and MRI imaging, and from a specialist surgical approach [19, 20].

Over the past decades, surgical treatment for UC has been refined to offer patients needing colectomy a better quality of life. Restorative proctocolectomy with ileal pouch-anal anastomosis (IPAA) is currently the gold standard procedure for most patients with UC requiring colectomy, offering them an unchanged body image without ileostomy and a preserved anal defecation and continence [8, 9, 17, 18].

However, despite general patient satisfaction, this procedure is associated with a significant long-term morbidity approaching 70 % after 10 years, and with a non-negligible (15 %) rate of pouch failure that leads to a permanent ileostomy. In the past, fluoroscopic pouchography using water-soluble contrast introduced through the loop ileostomy before its closure or retrogradely through the anus was performed to image possible IPAA-related complications [21, 22].

More recently, cross-sectional imaging has been increasingly employed at most referral centres. Knowledge of the surgical technique and of normal imaging appearance of the ileal "pouch" reservoir at pelvic CT and MRI is necessary to interpret postoperative studies requested by the surgeon when early complications are suspected [22, 23].

Although there are no clear recommendations on pouch surveillance, patients treated with proctocolectomy and IPAA need a close, prolonged, and individualized clinical and instrumental follow-up, due to the high incidence of pouch-related complications [8, 9, 17, 18]. In our experience, thanks to its limited invasiveness and diagnostic accuracy MRI has proved particularly useful to assess pouch-related disorders, and to distinguish uncomplicated pouchitis from pelvic sepsis, the latter needing surgical revision and pouch removal [23].

References

1. Stange EF, Travis SP, Vermeire S et al (2008) European evidence-based consensus on the diagnosis and management of ulcerative colitis: definitions and diagnosis. J Crohns Colitis 2:1–23
2. Dignass A, Eliakim R, Magro F et al (2012) Second European evidence-based consensus on the diagnosis and management of ulcerative colitis part 1: definitions and diagnosis. J Crohns Colitis 6:965–990
3. Kelvin FM, Oddson TA, Rice RP, Garbutt JT, Bradenham BP (1978) Double contrast barium enema in crohn's disease and ulcerative colitis. AJR Am J Roentgenol 131:207–213

4. Freeny PC (1986) Crohn's disease and ulcerative colitis. Evaluation with double-contrast barium examination and endoscopy. Postgrad Med 80:139–146, 149:152–136

5. Maccioni F, Colaiacomo MC, Parlanti S (2005) Ulcerative colitis: value of MR imaging. Abdom Imaging 30:584–592

6. Maccioni F (2010) Double-contrast magnetic resonance imaging of the small and large bowel: effectiveness in the evaluation of inflammatory bowel disease. Abdom Imaging 35:31–40

7. Patel B, Mottola J, Sahni VA et al (2012) MDCT assessment of ulcerative colitis: radiologic analysis with clinical, endoscopic, and pathologic correlation. Abdom Imaging 37:61–69

8. Travis SP, Stange EF, Lemann M et al (2008) European evidence-based consensus on the management of ulcerative colitis: current management. J Crohns Colitis 2:24–62

9. Dignass A, Lindsay JO, Sturm A et al (2012) Second European evidence-based consensus on the diagnosis and management of ulcerative colitis part 2: current management. J Crohns Colitis 6:991–1030

10. Hatoum OA, Spinelli KS, Abu-Hajir M et al (2005) Mesenteric venous thrombosis in inflammatory bowel disease. J Clin Gastroenterol 39:27–31

11. Saich R, Chapman R (2008) Primary sclerosing cholangitis, autoimmune hepatitis and overlap syndromes in inflammatory bowel disease. World J Gastroenterol 14:331–337

12. Nahon S, Cadranel JF, Chazouilleres O et al (2009) Liver and inflammatory bowel disease. Gastroenterol Clin Biol 33:370–381

13. Navaneethan U, Shen B (2010) Hepatopancreatobiliary manifestations and complications associated with inflammatory bowel disease. Inflamm Bowel Dis 16:1598–1619

14. Jackson CS, Fryer J, Danese S et al (2011) Mesenteric vascular thromboembolism in inflammatory bowel disease: a single center experience. J Gastrointest Surg 15:97–100

15. Lefevre A, Soyer P, Vahedi K et al (2011) Multiple intra-abdominal venous thrombosis in ulcerative colitis: role of MDCT for detection. Clin Imaging 35:68–72

16. Maconi G, Bolzacchini E, Dell'Era A et al (2012) Portal vein thrombosis in inflammatory bowel diseases: a single-center case series. J Crohns Colitis 6:362–367

17. Biancone L, Michetti P, Travis S et al (2008) European evidence-based consensus on the management of ulcerative colitis: special situations. J Crohns Colitis 2:63–92

18. Van Assche G, Dignass A, Bokemeyer B et al (2013) Second European evidence-based consensus on the diagnosis and management of ulcerative colitis part 3: special situations. J Crohns Colitis 7:1–33

19. Hamzaoglu I, Hodin RA (2005) Perianal problems in patients with ulcerative colitis. Inflamm Bowel Dis 11:856–859

20. Zabana Y, Van Domselaar M, Garcia-Planella E et al (2011) Perianal disease in patients with ulcerative colitis: a case-control study. J Crohns Colitis 5:338–341

21. Fazio VW, Ziv Y, Church JM et al (1995) Ileal pouch-anal anastomoses complications and function in 1005 patients. Ann Surg 222:120–127

22. Alfisher MM, Scholz FJ, Roberts PL, Counihan T (1997) Radiology of ileal pouch-anal anastomosis: normal findings, examination pitfalls, and complications. Radiographics 17:81–98 (discussion 98–89)

23. Tonolini M, Campari A, Bianco R (2011) Ileal pouch and related complications: spectrum of imaging findings with emphasis on MRI. Abdom Imaging 36:698–706

Medical Needs

2

Emilia Bareggi and Michela Monteleone

2.1 Introduction

Ulcerative colitis (UC) is a chronic inflammatory condition causing continuous mucosal inflammation of the colon, characterized by alternate periods of remission and relapse, affecting a variable extent of the large bowel, with a way of spreading from distal to proximal segments.

In clinical practice, normally we need some important information about disease that can settle some choices on patient management and therapy such as extent of inflammation, age and date of symptoms onset, disease activity and presence of intestinal or extraintestinal complications.

UC is classified according to disease extent, using the Montreal endoscopic classification: in proctitis, left-sided colitis up to the splenic flexure, and in extensive colitis, beyond the splenic flexure. This classification has important implications because it influences the patient's management and the choice of therapy. The extent of colitis influences the start and frequency of surveillance, being one of the risk factors for development of colorectal cancer: in left-sided and extensive colitis, endoscopic surveillance is generally recommended but no increased tumour risk is attributed to proctitis and these patients do not need surveillance.

Clinical disease activity is also divided into three groups: mild, moderate and severe. The definition of severity of disease is useful for clinical practice because it also influences the patient's management, treatment modality and necessity of none, oral, intravenous or surgical therapy [1].

The diagnosis can be made at any age, but most patients are diagnosed at a young age and these patients have often an aggressive disease. So it is important to consider that many young patients have to undergo repetitive imaging procedures during the variable course of disease and monitoring the response to treatment. Furthermore, the long duration of disease and aggressiveness of colitis are other risk factors for development of colorectal cancer and can influence the start of surveillance.

The presence of concomitant extraintestinal complications can also influence patient management.

Diagnosis of UC is based on a combination of medical history, clinical symptoms, laboratory tests and imaging data: no single imaging technique serves as a diagnostic gold standard for the diagnosis of UC.

Colonoscopy plays an extremely important, pivotal role in the diagnostic path, and management of ulcerative colitis, as with biopsies, it allows to define the presence and type of injury, as well as the extent of disease and the extent of histological involvement, information necessary

E. Bareggi (✉) · M. Monteleone
Department of Gastroenterology, "Luigi Sacco"
University Hospital, Via G.B. Grassi, 74, 20157
Milan, Italy
e-mail: bareggi.emilia@hsacco.it

M. Tonolini (ed.), *Imaging of Ulcerative Colitis*,
DOI: 10.1007/978-88-470-5409-7_2, © Springer-Verlag Italia 2014

to direct the choice of treatment. However, colonoscopy is an invasive procedure, not always accepted by patients and not devoid of complications.

As alternative to colonoscopy, various methods for assessing the level of inflammation of the colorectal mucosa have been proposed in recent years. Radiologic methods, thanks to technological development, are important tools for the diagnosis and evaluation of patients with ulcerative colitis.

The most used diagnostic imaging techniques are ultrasound (US), computed tomography (CT) and magnetic resonance (MR).

The clinician's method of choice is based on the technique, the information that allows to obtain and the clinical condition of the patient. They may not represent a valid alternative to endoscopy for now, but employed properly they can be considered complementary methods.

Cross-sectional diagnostic imaging is used in ulcerative colitis with a dual purpose: (1) to suggest the diagnosis in patients with suspected chronic inflammatory disease and (2) to gain useful information for the management of patients with known ulcerative colitis and, in particular, to assess the extent and activity of the disease or the presence of complications, mainly the neoplastic degeneration of mucosa at early stages [2].

The first step is to evaluate the clinical status of the patient, as an active disease precludes the use of invasive techniques. By contrast, in the case of mild or moderate disease, colonoscopy, CT or MR colonography (which have almost completely supplanted the barium enema) may be highly useful due to numerous findings that can highlight, in particular, the subtle definition of the alterations of the wall and the possibility of detecting extraintestinal alterations.

In addition, in case of suspicion of intestinal or extraintestinal complications, the radiologic methods find ample space in their diagnosis and staging. Therefore, the task of the clinician is to identify the most useful imaging method to make the diagnosis, whereas that of the radiologist is to

recognize and provide the clinician with information necessary for its decision [3].

This chapter reviews some of the common clinical situations that clinicians may face in patients with suspected or known UC, and discusses the information that is expected from the radiologist and the appropriate diagnostic imaging modalities.

2.2   Mild or Moderate Ulcerative Colitis

B.M, a 56-year-old man, complained of diarrhoea (3–4 bloody stools/day) for more than 6 weeks, associated with rectal bleeding and rectal urgency, with normal temperatures and no abdominal pain. Laboratory investigations showed normal markers of chronic inflammation (C-reactive protein CRP, erythrocyte sedimentation rate ESR) and normal full blood count. He was an ex-smoker (20 cigarettes/day, stopped at least 1 year ago) and had no other previous important pathologies. He underwent colonoscopy, which demonstrated the presence of a hyperemic and granular mucosa, with erosions of rectum and distal sigma and normal appearance of proximal colon. Histologic examination could establish the suspect of ulcerative colitis in distal samples.

Which information does the clinician need in this patient? What investigations should the patient undergo to arrive at a correct diagnosis and correct management?

For the clinician it is necessary to identify some basic parameters that will allow him to determine the most appropriate therapy and future behaviour: establish a correct diagnosis considering most common causes of chronic diarrhoea, evaluation of extent of disease, activity, severity of inflammation, presence of complications and post-treatment modifications.

Following ECCO guidelines, colonoscopy (preferably with ileoscopy and segmental biopsies including the rectum) is the preferred procedure to establish the diagnosis and extent of disease.

The differential diagnosis should be done between UC and acute inflammatory conditions such as infectious colitis, diverticular sigmoiditis and ischaemic lesions, the last one eventually requiring ultrasonographic study of mesenteric circulation.

Obviously, the initial diagnosis of UC requires the elimination of infectious causes of symptomatic colitis: stool specimens should be cultured for common pathogens and fresh stool samples should be examined for parasites [1].

Depending on extension and activity of disease, the severity of symptoms (such as diarrhoea, rectal blood loss, abdominal pain and fever) can vary, and laboratory parameters of the acute phase response (CRP, ESR and faecal calprotectin) may be normal or abnormal.

Rectosigmoid involvement is present in almost all patients at endoscopy: approximately 40–50 % of patients have disease limited to the rectum and recto-sigma, 30–40 % have a left-sided colitis and 20 % a total colitis.

Proximal spread of the disease, from the rectum to the cecum, occurs in continuity without areas of uninvolved mucosa. However, macroscopical sparing of the rectum has been described in children prior to treatment. In adults, normal or patchy inflammation of the rectum, is likely to be due to topical therapy, but endoscopic biopsies from mucosa with a normal appearance are usually abnormal.

The mucosa may appear normal when disease is in remission, whereas in mild and moderate disease the mucosa is erythematous, oedematous, of granular appearance, with loss of normal vascular pattern. In more severe cases, the mucosa is ulcerated and haemorrhagic. In long-standing disease, the mucosa may appear atrophic-cicatricial and inflammatory pseudo-polyps may be present as a result of epithelial regeneration.

In UC, histological changes are limited to the mucosa and superficial submucosa with deeper layers being unaffected, except in fulminant colitis. The major changes include distortion of crypt architecture or crypt atrophy, mucin depletion, Paneth cell metaplasia and infiltrate in lamina propria of basal plasma cells.

However, since the disease is confined to the inner layers of the bowel wall, endoscopy with biopsies alone may be sufficient to detect and assess the extent and activity of the disease in UC. In this context, the role of cross-sectional imaging methods may be marginal, although they may be useful in presence of rectal sparing or atypical symptoms that can induce to diagnostic mistakes. Fundamental in these cases is, when possible, the differentiation of ulcerative colitis from Crohn's disease, important from prognostic and therapeutic points of view.

In some cases, associated with colonoscopy, bowel ultrasound can be useful as complementary diagnostic technique to help differential diagnosis and it has the advantage of being non-invasive, easy to perform without prior preparation, easily repeatable and inexpensive [4].

Imaging procedures such as CT or MRI colonography (enema CT with introduction of air or water and iodinated contrast media intravenously) can allow the simultaneous evaluation of the lumen, the gut wall and extraluminal changes, permitting a great panoramic study of abdomen and for this reason they are therefore becoming the investigation of choice in case of incomplete colonoscopy [5].

Definition of extension of colitis has a great importance to establish the first line therapy, which can be a topical therapy in proctitis, in the form of suppositories or enemas, or a systemic therapy often combined with topical therapy, in left-sided colitis or extensive colitis [1].

2.3 Severe Disease

V.M. is a 32-year-old woman with a 6-month diagnosis of left-sided ulcerative colitis, presenting at emergency room referring 7–8 bloody stools/day, nausea and vomiting; at physical examination she presented tachycardia and cutaneous pallor, with severe tenderness in the left abdominal quadrants. Laboratory analysis showed marked elevated values of CRP and

ESR, thrombocytosis and severe anemia (7.8 g/dl). Since initial diagnosis, she had undergone one cycle of systemic steroid therapy at high dose, with initial but not complete benefits and reappearance of symptoms at tapering of steroid.

From one week before her arrival at hospital, she restarted steroid therapy at high dose (methylprednisolone 60 mg/die), without any benefit.

During recovery, she underwent plain abdominal radiograph that excluded perforation or colonic dilatation and sigmoidoscopy, which demonstrated the presence of markedly inflamed mucosa in the explored tract, spontaneously bleeding and with deep ulcerations. After excluding *Clostridium difficile* superinfection with analysis of stool sample and cytomegalovirus (CMV) on histology and serological research of DNA, clinicians started intravenous Cyclosporine at dose 2.5 mg/kg/die.

At the end of the fifth day of intravenous immunosuppressant therapy, after a period of apparent benefit, she had the reappearance of important bleeding with severe hypotension; a plain abdominal radiograph, and bowel US showed dilatation of right-sided colon and ileum. So the decision of clinicians was to subject the patient to urgent colectomy.

Which are symptoms of severe attack and which approach must the clinician take?

Clinically bloody stool frequency, systemic symptoms such as elevation of body temperature and presence of tachycardia, are good predictors of outcome.

At diagnosis, every patient must undergo laboratory analysis: anemia, elevation of laboratory tests of inflammation, electrolytes alteration and hypoalbuminemia can be present. Stool samples for microbiological testing, including *Cl. difficile*, are necessary and serological testing for CMV is recommended in case of severe or refractory disease, especially in immunosuppressed patients.

A plain abdominal radiograph is recommended in the initial assessment of the patient and should be performed not only to exclude the presence of complications, such as perforation or toxic megacolon (colonic dilatation >5 cm), but

also to estimate the extent of disease and predict the response to treatment. The distribution of faecal residue is an indirect sign of disease, since the proximal extent of disease grossly corresponds to the distal distribution of faecal residue. Besides, persistent colonic distension in severe UC correlates with poor response to therapy and with higher rate of toxic megacolon [1]. Incidence of toxic colitis in UC is between 6 and 13 %, with a high risk of mortality.

An active disease must be confirmed by sigmoidoscopy as a first line procedure, since more invasive procedures can be dangerous and are contraindicated. It helps to confirm diagnosis and to exclude infections, particularly with CMV.

Also, the intestinal ultrasound in this phase may have a role in identifying and characterizing the thickening of the colonic walls, mesenteric fat hypertrophy and presence of lymph nodes, and it plays a supportive role when complications are clinically suspected; toxic megacolon should be suspected when US shows marked decrease in thickness (<2 mm) of the colonic wall, associated with dilatation (>6 cm) of the colon, and increased fluid and dilation of the ileal loops [6, 7].

Contrast-enhanced abdominal CT can be performed when the evaluation of extraluminal alterations and exclusion of possible complications is necessary (perforation, colonic dilatation or stenosis), directing the subsequent course of treatment.

In these patients, the clinical approach and consequently the therapeutic one, after the exclusion of possible superinfection or complications, must be multidisciplinary: systemic steroid therapy, intravenous immunosuppressant or biological therapy are possible medical therapies, but when disease becomes refractory to conventional therapies or in case of complications, surgical colectomy becomes necessary

Indications to perform colectomy mainly include toxic colitis, acute perforation (in presence or not of toxic colitis), severe rectal bleeding, which can arise in 50 % of toxic megacolon, bowel occlusion as a consequence of a stenosis, dysplasia and cancer.

2.4 Neoplastic Degeneration

A.L. is a 63-year-old patient, with a history of ulcerative colitis (pancolitis) for 18 years, on maintenance therapy with Sulfasalazin for correlated articular symptoms. During endoscopic surveillance, in a phase of remission of disease, he was subjected to removal of two small polyps of the ascending colon, histologically compatible with tubular adenomas with low-grade dysplasia. The following chromoendoscopy permitted to find a suspected flat area in ascending colon that histologically resulted in an area of low-grade dysplasia. After discussion with the patient about the risks, benefits, and limits of surveillance and after surgical consultation, it was decided that colectomy would be the best choice, because it could completely eradicate the risk of colorectal cancer.

One of the main complications of UC is neoplastic degeneration, a condition with an incidence highly dependent on the time and extent of the disease. Eden and co. in a meta-analysis of 194 studies estimated that the cumulative probability of colorectal cancer (CRC) in patients with ulcerative colitis, regardless of the extent of disease, was 2 % after 10 years of disease, 8 % after 20 years and 18 % after 30 years of disease [8].

Risk factors for CRC in IBD include disease duration >8 years, disease extension with both macro and microscopic assessment (pancolitis > left-sided colitis > proctitis), concomitant Primary Sclerosing Cholangitis (PSC), family history of CRC in a first-degree relative, more severe or persistent endoscopic activity, pseudopolyposis, histological activity and stricture. CRC risk is not increased in patients with UC limited to the rectum.

Dysplasia is considered the best marker of cancer risk in UC. The clinical management depends on the endoscopic and histological findings by an expert pathologist.

Since dysplastic changes in colonic mucosa is associated with an increased risk of CRC in UC, surveillance colonoscopy programmes have been developed with the aim of reducing morbidity and mortality due to CRC. For this reason in all patients with UC a screening colonoscopy could be carried out 8–10 years after the beginning of symptoms in order to assess the patients' individual risk profile, that dictates next surveillance colonoscopy intervals.

After the screening colonoscopy, endoscopic surveillance should be performed periodically with a frequency not yet well-defined.

According to ECCO guidelines 2012, the endoscopic surveillance should be carried out according to the risk of CRC every 1–2 years in patients with high risk (more than 3 risk factors) and every 3–4 years in patients with low risk (less than 2 risk factors). In cases with concurrent primary sclerosing cholangitis, surveillance colonoscopy should be carried out yearly from the diagnosis of PSC. In proctitis, endoscopic surveillance is not required [9, 10].

Chromoendoscopy is the procedure of choice for surveillance, but it needs a trained endoscopist and when it is not possible, random biopsies every 10 cm on every quadrant, are recommended.

Therapeutic recommendations for management of dysplasia, conducing to colectomy or increased surveillance, are based on macroscopic and microscopic patterns of dysplasia; macroscopically, dysplasia can be flat or raised. Raised dysplasia can be adenoma-like (endoscopically resectable), non-adenoma-like (endoscopically non-resectable) or as sporadic adenoma. Histologically, dysplasia can be divided into low-grade dysplasia (LGD) and high-grade dysplasia (HGD). Patients with HGD have higher risk of progression to colorectal cancer. In presence of flat high-grade dysplasia, confirmed by a second pathologist, colectomy is the treatment of choice, but in case of low-grade dysplasia there is uncertainty in all guidelines. In case of sporadic adenomas, patients should be subjected to polypectomy and regular surveillance. Finding of adenoma-like dysplasia inside involved colon requires polypectomy, confirmation of absence of flat dysplasia and negative margins, and increased surveillance. In case of non-adenoma-like dysplasia colectomy is always indicated.

There is evidence that cancers tend to be detected at earlier stages in patients who undergo surveillance, and these patients have a correspondingly better prognosis [11].

Furthermore, a colonic stricture in long-standing ulcerative colitis correlates with an increased risk for colorectal carcinoma and requires careful histological assessment with multiple biopsies. If colonoscopy is incomplete, it is important to assess the mucosal pattern proximal to the stricture, as well as wall infiltration and extraintestinal abnormalities; CT or MR colonography have become the investigations of choice in this situation.

Therapy with 5-aminosalicylates is considered to reduce the risk of colorectal cancer in patients with UC, so this therapy must be considered for all patients, except for those with isolated proctitis.

2.5   Primary Sclerosing Cholangitis

C.Z. is a 22-year-old patient, with a diagnosis of ulcerative colitis when he was twelve years old. Clinical history was characterized by initial development of steroid dependence, after 1 year from diagnosis, and rapid introduction of immunosuppressant therapy with thiopurines, which was prolonged for 5 years and then stopped for persistent clinical remission, maintaining only clinical observation.

He arrived at the attention of the gastroenterologist for occasional finding at laboratory tests of elevated serum liver tests (aminotransaminase twice the upper normal limit) and particularly of cholestatic enzymes (marked elevation of gamma glutamyl transpherase and alkaline phosphatase), with normality of other laboratory analysis. He referred no symptoms, except for the presence of a moderate asthenia and showed an abdominal US that documented the dilatation (9 mm) of the main bile duct, with thickened walls.

After exclusion of infective causes and autoimmune liver disorders, he was subjected to a magnetic resonance cholangiography (MRCP) which showed a diffuse irregularity of the common bile duct and intrahepatic small ducts, characterized by the presence of narrowed and dilatated tracts, compatible with an inflammatory biliary disease.

A therapy with ursodeoxycholic acid was promptly started and he was sent to a programme of annual endoscopic surveillance for detection of colorectal cancer.

PSC is a chronic cholestatic disease characterized by inflammation and fibrosis of intra and extrahepatic bile ducts, which leads to progressive obliteration of the bile ducts and finally to development of secondary biliary cirrhosis.

The frequency of PSC in patients with IBD is reported in the range 2.5 %–7.5 %.

Its aetiology is unknown and the majority of patients are asymptomatic at diagnosis, presenting only alteration of predominantly obstructive liver enzymes at routine laboratory examinations. However, some patients can have fatigue, or symptoms correlated to biliary obstruction as fever, jaundice, pruritus and weight loss.

So patients with IBD and associated cholestatic liver test elevations , with negative serological tests for infectious or autoimmune hepatic disorders, should be assessed for PSC: MRCP is now established as the first line diagnostic test for PSC. When MRCP is normal, in case of strong suspect, it is useful to perform a liver biopsy to evaluate a predominant small duct involvement.

ERCP remains the procedure of choice only for therapeutic relief of biliary strictures and for evaluation of strictures to exclude malignancy.

Currently, there is no effective medical therapy for reducing or preventing disease progression; ursodeoxycholic acid (UDCA), at doses between 10 and 15 mg/kg/day, is associated with biochemical and histological improvement, but without important survival differences with respect to placebo.

In advanced disease with liver failure, the only effective therapy is liver transplantation, but recurrence of disease in transplanted liver occurs in approximately 20–25 % of patients after 5–10 years post-transplant [9, 12].

It is fundamental to arrive at a diagnosis as soon as possible, since PSC increases the risk of both cholangiocarcinoma (CCA) and colorectal carcinoma (CRC). Patients with UC and PSC have a fourfold higher risk of colorectal cancer and for this reason it is necessary, from diagnosis of PSC, to perform annual screening colonoscopy (in transplanted patients too).

There is no screening programme to detect early CCA. Current practice includes the use of serum carbohydrate antigen 19.9 and cross-sectional imaging examinations and in case of significant changes in one or both tests, ERCP and brush cytology or biopsy are necessary to detect CCA. Therapeutic options are limited and these patients continue to have poor 5-year survival rates; patients with unresectable CCA can be candidate to liver transplantation after a multimodal approach using radiotherapy and chemotherapy.

Therapy with UDCA at standard doses, like aminosalicylate agents (5-ASA), seems to be related to a reduced risk of colorectal cancer in UC, but not all studies seem to confirm this potential benefit and prospective studies are necessary [12].

2.6   Pouch Disorders

V.A., 51-years old, in September 2005 underwent urgent chirurgical restorative proctocolectomy, with temporary cutaneous ileostomy for ulcerative colitis not responsive to conventional therapies and complicated with severe rectal bleeding. After some months of good clinical conditions, he underwent creation of ileal-pouch reservoir and pouch-anal anastomosis (IPAA).

At his next clinical visit, he referred several stool evacuations in a day, also nocturnal, sometimes with presence of blood, without any benefits from the use of anti-diarrhoic drugs. Pouchscopy showed diffuse erythema, oedema and friability of mucosa, covered with multiple aftoid ulcerations and histological examination demonstrating a non-specific acute and chronic

inflammation, with focal superficial ulcerations and crypt abscesses.

He soon started cyclical antibiotic therapies with ciprofloxacin and metronidazole, without benefits.

Next, he referred increased stool evacuations (>10/day) with rectal bleeding, abdominal pain, soiling and loss of weight of 5–6 kg in 3 months, with moderate elevation of inflammatory indexes. So he underwent another pouchscopy that showed great friability, marked hyperemia and oedema of the mucosa, with serpiginous ulcerations and normal ileal limb afferent to the pouch. Histological examination confirmed the presence of a non-specific acute and chronic inflammation.

After other cyclical antibiotic and probiotic therapies, prolonged for at least 1 year, without any clinical or endoscopic benefit and after exclusion of *Cl. difficile* or cytomegalovirus infection, he was candidate to biological therapy for refractory pouchitis.

He was subjected to six infusions of Inflix-imab at a dose of 5 mg/kg, also with reduced intervals between infusions and at increasing dosage with no clinical or endoscopic answer; for this reason, it was decided to stop biological therapy and to introduce a last therapeutic attempt with Budesonide at a dose of 9 mg/kg/die for 2 months, that was stopped by himself for worsening of clinical conditions. The next endoscopic evaluation demonstrated persistent active inflammation of the pouch reservoir and he was candidate to pouch removal and permanent ileostomy.

Proctocolectomy with ileal-pouch-anal anastomosis (IPAA) is the procedure of choice for most patients with UC requiring colectomy, because of disease refractory to medical therapy or dysplastic changes.

IPAA is associated with a significant long-term morbidity approaching 70 % after 10 years and with a high rate of pouch failure leading to removal and permanent ileostomy.

After surgery, clinical and instrumental follow-up is recommended for the significant incidence of pouch-related complications such as pouchitis, anastomotic leakages and pelvic abscess collections, perianal and anovaginal fistulas, anal stenosis and small bowel obstructions [13].

Pouchitis, the most common complication of IPAA in patients with UC, is a non-specific inflammation of the ileal reservoir, whose aetiology remains unknown. Its frequency is related to the duration of follow-up, occurring in up to 50 % of patients 10 years after IPAA. Probably an interaction between the host immune response and the pouch microbiota plays a role in its occurrence.

Extensive UC, PSC, being a non-smoker and the regular use of NSAID, are possible risk factors for pouchitis.

Diagnosis is based on symptoms and characteristic endoscopic and histological features.

The activity score proposed for diagnosis of pouchitis (Pouchitis Disease Activity Index, PDAI) is based on three parameters: clinical, endoscopical and histological.

Symptoms include increased stool frequency, abdominal pain, urgency, tenesmus and pelvic discomfort. Rectal bleeding, faecal incontinence or extraintestinal manifestations are rare.

Pouchscopy with biopsy should be performed in patients with symptoms compatible with pouchitis, in order to confirm the diagnosis. Endoscopic examination completed by histological examination of biopsies is essential to define the presence of pouchitis and to exclude the diagnosis of "irritable pouch syndrome," in which symptoms do not correspond to a real endoscopic and/or histological inflammation.

Endoscopic aspects of pouchitis are mucosal oedema, erythema, granularity, friability, spontaneous or contact bleeding, erosions and ulcerations; ulcerations along the staple line are not strictly indicative of the presence of pouchitis. Histological finding is normally a non-specific acute inflammation, with crypt abscesses and ulcerations, in association with a chronic inflammatory infiltrate.

Depending on duration of symptoms, pouchitis can be divided into acute or chronic.

In acute pouchitis, antibiotics as ciprofloxacin or metronidazole are the first line treatment, often resulting in a rapid response; also highly concentrated probiotic preparations have been effective in the treatment of mildly pouchitis and in maintaining remission or preventing pouchitis.

Chronic pouchitis (duration of symptoms >4 weeks) normally requires long-term treatment with a combination of two antibiotics or oral budesonide; in rare cases pouchitis can be refractory to medical therapy and this is a common cause for pouch failure. In this case it is important to consider different diagnoses, first of all a misdiagnosed Crohn's disease, superinfection with CMV or *clostridium difficile*, ileal-pouch or anal-pouch strictures, anatomical disorders or irritable pouch syndrome.

Immunomodulator therapy with infliximab can be effective in some patients with chronic refractory pouchitis.

Complications of pouchitis include abscesses, fistulae, stenosis of ileal-pouch or pouch-anal anastomosis, and adenocarcinoma of the pouch, the last one occurring principally in patients who underwent colectomy for dysplasia or carcinoma [9].

Strictures may develop as a complication of surgical techniques. Perianal fistulae are usually secondary to stenosis of the pouch-anal anastomosis, or the result of a chronic inflammation or of an unrevealed CD.

Pelvic MRI has been reported as a very accurate modality for the assessment of possible pouch-related complications, thanks to its diagnostic accuracy, panoramic view, excellent detection of abscesses, fistulas and inflammatory activity. MRI is feasible even in patients with anal stenosis or pain, does not require special bowel preparation, has limited invasiveness, and is particularly beneficial in young patients, often needing repeated studies [14].

When is endoscopic surveillance in patients with IPAA suggested?

There are no sure indications on execution of endoscopic surveillance after proctocolectomy with IPAA; endoscopy is always indicated in cases of clinical suspect of pouchitis, while the need for endoscopic surveillance of dysplasia or CRC is uncertain. Normally, surveillance of dysplasia/CRC is not indicated except in cases of concomitant presence of high risk of CRC or significant residual rectal mucosa (patients with extended cuff).

A proctoscopy is suggested annually in presence of ileal-rectal anastomosis.

Endoscopic surveillance is also recommended in patients with chronic pouchitis, or with an increased risk of colorectal cancer for concomitant primary sclerosing cholangitis, family history or genetic predisposition, or in patients that required colectomy for dysplastic changes or neoplastic degeneration; in these cases pouchscopy must be performed at least annually.

A further indication to perform an endoscopic examination of IPAA is represented by those patients with clinical suspicion of Crohn's disease, due to its different prognostic and therapeutic implications.

References

1. Dignass A, Eliakim R, Magro F, Maaser C, Chowers Y, Geboes K, Mantzaris G, Walter R, Colombel JF, Vermeire S, Travis S, Lindsay JO, Assche GV (2012) Second European evidence-based Consensus on the diagnosis and management of ulcerative colitis: definitions and diagnosis. Ecco Guidelines (Edition 2012)
2. Pompili G, Franceschelli G, Massiroli C, Villa A, Cornalba GP (2006) Radiologia convenzionale: è ancora utile e quando? In IBD Year Book 2006. Nomos Edizioni, pp 51–61
3. Maconi G, Greco S, Radice E, Ardizzone S, Colombo E, Bianchi Porro G (2006) Nuove metodiche diagnostiche per immagini nella colite ulcerosa. In IBD Year Book 2006. Nomos Edizioni, pp 63–76
4. Strobel D, Goertz R, Bernatik T (2011) Diagnostics in inflammatory bowel disease: ultrasound. World J Gastroenterol 17(27):3192–3197
5. Gee MS, Harisinghani MG (2011) MRI in patients with inflammatory bowel disease. J Magn Reson Imaging 33(3):527–534
6. Maconi G, Sampietro GM, Ardizzone S et al (2004) US detection of toxic megacolon in inflammatory bowel diseases. Dig Dis Sci 49:138–142
7. Maconi G, Ardizzone S, Parente F, Bianchi Porro G (1999) Ultrasonography in the evaluation of extension, activity, and follow-up of ulcerative colitis. Scand J Gastroenterol 34:1103–1107
8. Eaden JA, Abrams KR, Mayberry JF (2001) The risk of colorectal cancer in ulcerative colitis: a metanalysis. Gut 48:526–535
9. Van Assche G, Dignass A, Bokemeyer B et al (2013) Second European evidence-based consensus on the diagnosis and management of ulcerative colitis part 3: Special situations. J Crohns Colitis 7:1–33
10. Dyson JK, Rutter MD (2012) Colorectal cancer in inflammatory bowel disease: what is the real magnitude of the risk? World J Gastroenterol 18(29):3839–3848
11. Neuman H, Vieth M, Langner C, Neurath MF, Mudter J (2011) Cancer risk in IBD: how to diagnose and how to manage DALM and ALM. World J Gastroenterol 17(27):3184–3191
12. Eaton JE, Talwalkar JA (2013) Primary sclerosing cholangitis: current and future management strategies. Current hepatitis reports. Springer Science + Business Media New York 2013; 10.1007/s11901-012-0155-1
13. Tonolini M, Campari A, Bianco R (2011) Ileal pouch and related complications: spectrum of imaging findings with emphasis on MRI. Abdom Imaging 36:698–706
14. Tonolini M (2013) Ulcerative colitis and ileal pouch surgery. Imaging of perianal inflammatory diseases. Springer-Verlag Italia, pp 177–183

Intestinal Ultrasound in Ulcerative Colitis

3

Cristina Bezzio, Federica Furfaro, Michela Monteleone
and Giovanni Maconi

3.1 Introduction

Endoscopy is the method of choice in the diagnosis and in assessing extent and severity of ulcerative colitis (UC). In ulcerative colitis, inflammatory lesions are confined to the mucosa and have a predictable spreading involving mainly the rectum that is difficult to assess by conventional imaging methods, including transabdominal ultrasound.

However, the scientific literature has demonstrated that intestinal ultrasound is a reliable diagnostic tool to detect disease extension and activity in ulcerative colitis. It may provide important information if endoscopy is incomplete or contraindicated, and may suggest the outcome of disease after therapy.

3.2 Technique of Examination

Sonographic investigation of the gastrointestinal tract is performed using conventional ultrasonographic probes: convex 3.5–5 MHz probe, to have an overview of the gastrointestinal tract and high resolution 4–13 MHz linear or microconvex probe for a detailed visualization of the bowel wall. Lower frequencies are useful for the examination of deep abdominal structures and higher frequencies for superficial parts. The focus and gain of the instrument should be adjusted to optimize image resolution. Tissue harmonic imaging (THI) may improve the visualization of the features of the bowel wall, the luminal content and peri-intestinal findings, such as free fluid, mesenteric lymph nodes and mesenteric fat changes [1].

It is preferable to perform the bowel ultrasound in fasting condition, because the intake of a large quantity of liquid meals and water just before bowel ultrasound in some instances may mimic partial small bowel obstruction (e.g. due to adhesions) and malabsorption (e.g. celiac disease), hampering a correct diagnosis and the exclusion of these conditions. However, the fasting state is not mandatory (e.g. in acute abdomen, bowel ultrasound may be of value despite feeding condition).

Patients are examined in supine position but, if necessary, they may be turned on the left or right side or put in an upright position, to move the bowel and its content, to avoid the interference of gas and optimize the visualization of the features of bowel walls. Routine bowel evaluation usually should be systematically performed, e.g. starting from hypogastrium or left iliac fossa (i.e. from the sigmoid colon) and then continuing to examine the colon, terminal ileum,

C. Bezzio · F. Furfaro · M. Monteleone
Gastroenterology Unit, Department of Biomedical
and Clinical Sciences, L. Sacco University Hospital,
Milan, Italy

G. Maconi (✉)
Gastroenterology Unit, Department of Biomedical
and Clinical Sciences, L. Sacco University Hospital,
Via G.B. Grassi, 74, 20157 Milan, Italy
e-mail: giovanni.maconi@unimi.it

M. Tonolini (ed.), *Imaging of Ulcerative Colitis*,
DOI: 10.1007/978-88-470-5409-7_3, © Springer-Verlag Italia 2014

appendix and small bowel, up to the stomach. However, other examination sequences may be valid provided that the whole gut is assessed. In patients with acute abdominal pain, in particular when it is well localized, the bowel examination should be started from the maximum pain area.

The examination is performed using graded compression technique. This is useful to shift intraluminal gas and improve visualization of the posterior parts of the bowel, in particular the anatomical structures in the lower quadrants of the abdomen such as appendix, terminal ileum, caecum and sigmoid colon [2].

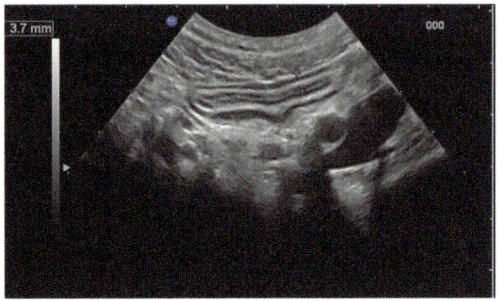

Fig. 3.2 Transversal ultrasonographic section of sigmoid colon in patient with quiescent ulcerative colitis. The stratified echopattern of the bowel wall is preserved and the thickness is within the normal values

3.3   Ultrasonographic Features

The ultrasonographic features of ulcerative colitis are bowel wall thickening, alterations of the bowel wall echo pattern and loss of haustra coli. Also, perivisceral manifestations can be observed such as mesenteric hypertrophy and enlarged lymph nodes.

The degree of bowel wall thickening in ulcerative colitis depends on the activity of the disease, being greater in active disease. In particular, in active ulcerative colitis patients, ultrasound frequently reveals thickened bowel walls, usually >4 mm, frequently ranging from 5 to 7 mm, but rarely >10 mm [3] (Fig. 3.1). By contrast, in the quiescent phase of the disease the

bowel thickening is usually normal (<4 mm) (Fig. 3.2).

In active ulcerative colitis, the thickness of the bowel wall is usually homogeneous and continuous, circumferential and symmetrical. It predominates in the left colon, it is easily detectable in the hypogastrium and extends throughout the entire colon in extensive colitis and in pancolitis.

In active and extensive disease, the bowel wall usually shows a stratified echopattern with loss of haustra coli. In acute colitis, the thickening involves the submucosa which may also appear slightly hypoechoic and dyshomogeneous, sometimes with loss of stratification and increased vascularity at colour Dopper. The muscularis propria, normally imaged as an external hypoechoic line, is preserved, and therefore the external profiles of the colonic wall in ulcerative colitis are usually linear and regular. Unlike Crohn's disease, ulcerations are usually superficial and not detectable by ultrasound and therefore in mild to moderate active ulcerative colitis, the inner layers of the colonic wall are usually regular. However, severe ulcerative colitis is characterized by markedly thickened and hypoechoic bowel walls (Fig. 3.3), sometimes with irregular inner layer and small linear hyperechoic spots representing deep penetrating ulcers of the submucosa. The bowel ultrasound can also suggest the presence of toxic megacolon when severely thickened and hypoechoic bowel wall in the left colon,

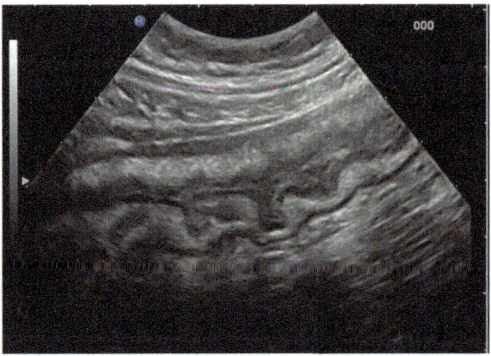

Fig. 3.1 Longitudinal section of descending colon in patient with *left*-sided active ulcerative colitis shows thickened bowel walls characterized by stratified echopattern and absence of haustra coli

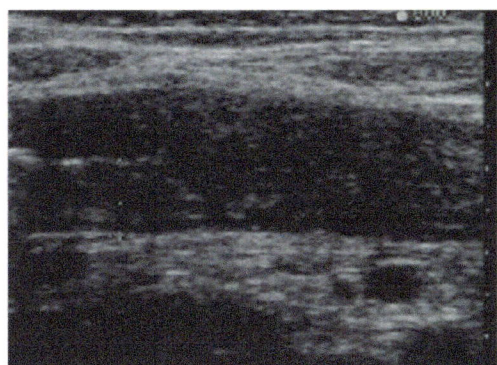

Fig. 3.3 Longitudinal ultrasonographic section of transverse colon in patients with severe ulcerative colitis showing thickened and hypoechoic bowel wall

associated with marked dilatation (>6 cm) of the transverse colon characterized by decrease in bowel wall thickness (<2 mm), and presence of increased fluid and dilation of the ileal loops, are

found (Fig. 3.4a and b) [4]. However, it should be acknowledged that ultrasound plays only a supportive role in this clinical context, which is still marginal in comparison to the plain abdominal radiography that is the reference investigation.

In quiescent ulcerative colitis, in particular in patients with previous several recurrences, as well as in some cases with mild inflammation, the colonic wall shows normal or only slight thickening with a predominant echogenic submucosa contrasting with the hypoechoic inner mucosa and outer muscularis (Fig. 3.5).

In ulcerative colitis patients with pseudopolyposis, small echogenic hypoechoic nodules may be observed at the surface of the mucosa (Fig. 3.6). These may be isolated and well appreciable into the fluid-filled intestinal lumen, also by using hydrocolonic sonography. Extensive pseudopolyposis appears as an increased and inhomogeneous thickness of the bowel wall (up to 15 mm), without the typical bowel wall stratification (also in quiescent ulcerative colitis), markedly irregular internal margins and/or as a dilated incompressible bowel with echogenic inhomogeneous content. The colour Doppler can be used to obtain confirmation of

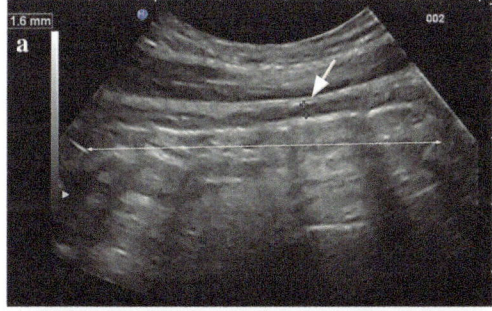

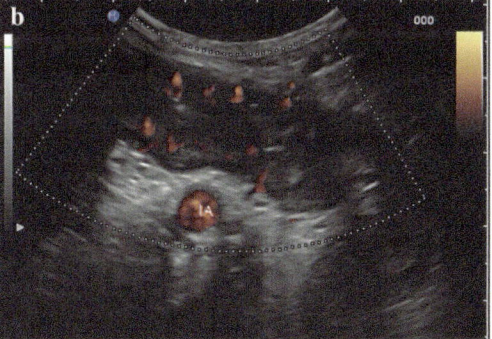

Fig. 3.4 Ultrasonographic findings in ulcerative colitis patient with impending toxic megacolon. **a** Thin hypoechoic bowel wall (*short arrow*) and dilated transverse colon (*long arrow*). **b** Longitudinal section of the sigmoid colon of the same patient showing thickened hypoechoic and hypervascularized bowel walls. IA, iliac artery

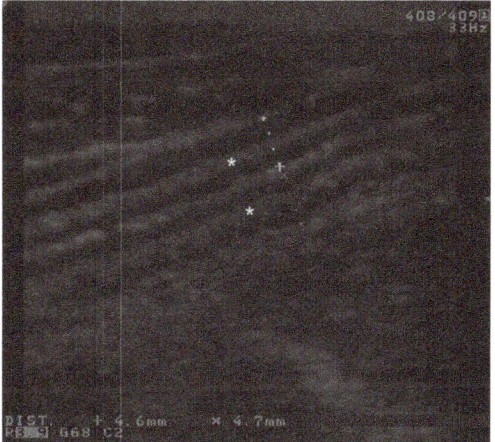

Fig. 3.5 Longitudinal ultrasonographic section of descending colon in patient with quiescent ulcerative colitis showing slight thickening of the bowel wall with preserved stratified echopattern and predominant echogenic submucosa (*asterisks*)

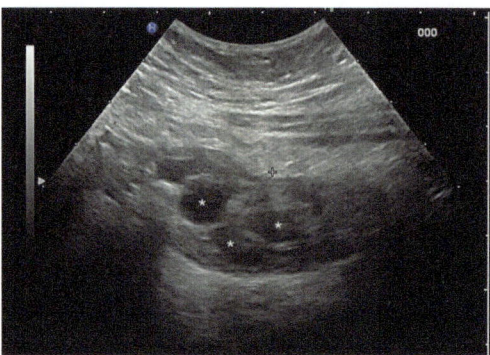

Fig. 3.6 Ulcerative colitis patients with pseudopolyposis. Longitudinal scan of the descending colon showing small echogenic hypoechoic nodules (*asterisks*) within the lumen

the pseudopolypoid nature of the intestinal content, assessing the blood flow within the echogenic material.

3.4　Diagnostic Accuracy

Bowel ultrasound has been demonstrated to be a reliable tool for diagnostic purposes, to assess disease extension and activity in ulcerative colitis, thus providing important information if endoscopy is incomplete or contraindicated, and also to predict the outcome of disease after therapy (Table 3.1).

Table 3.1 Indications and potential usefulness of bowel ultrasound in UC

Early evaluation of patients with suspected ulcerative colitis
Evaluation of extension
Assessment of activity
Assessment of response to therapy
Long-term prediction of outcome (relapse/remission)
Diagnosis of abdominal complications
–Toxic megacolon
–Pseudopolyposis
Differential diagnosis in chronic inflammatory colitis

3.4.1　Detection of Ulcerative Colitis and Assessment of Disease Activity

The studies carried out in adults, which have adopted the bowel wall thickness >4 mm as criterium for abnormality, have shown that transabdominal ultrasound has a median of 76 % (range: 53–89 %) in detecting ulcerative colitis [5–12]. The sensitivity in assessing ulcerative colitis is lower than that reported to assess other inflammatory bowel diseases, such as Crohn's disease or diverticulitis. This may be explained by the fact that inactive ulcerative colitis or disease characterized by mild inflammation has frequently normal bowel wall thickening (<4 mm) and when the disease activity is confined to the rectum, it is difficult to assess by transabdominal ultrasound .

Several studies have shown that the degree of bowel wall thickening correlates well with clinical activity [7, 8, 13–17], biochemical (namely C-reactive protein and erythrocyte sedimentation rate values) [14, 15, 18], endoscopic [14, 16, 18, 19] and scintigraphic activity [13] of ulcerative colitis.

A few studies have also shown that other ultrasonographic features, such as the loss of bowel wall stratification (hypoechoic echopattern) [9] or the increased bowel wall vascularity [20], may correlate with the clinical and endoscopic activity of ulcerative colitis.

3.4.2　Evaluation the Anatomical Extension

Bowel ultrasound has been proved to be of value in evaluating the anatomical extension of the inflammation during disease flare-up. In particular, the technique has a very high sensitivity in detecting left-sided colitis, although it has low sensitivity in identifying proctitis [10]. For these reasons, bowel ultrasound may be a valid alternative to invasive procedures in assessing the extension of ulcerative colitis, provided that the disease is active (e.g. bowel examination should be performed only during flare-up of the disease) and is not limited to the rectum (e.g. bowel examination may be negative in patients presenting without diarrhoea and only with rectal bleeding).

3.4.3 Response to Therapy and Outcome

Bowel ultrasound may evaluate the response to medical treatment in active ulcerative colitis and predict relapses of the disease [13, 14]. In severe ulcerative colitis, it has been shown that the absence of significant decrement in wall thickness from baseline, shortly after a course of therapy (high-dose steroid therapy or cytapheresis), is associated with a high risk of endoscopic relapse at 1 year [19–22].

The vascularity of the inferior mesenteric artery and superior mesenteric artery, assessed by Doppler sonography, has been also shown to be well correlated with clinical and endoscopic activity. Indeed, several studies have shown that mean velocity is significantly reduced, and pulsatility and resistance indexes of these arteries are increased compared to those in control subjects [23–28]. This suggests their potential usefulness in the evaluation of inflammation of the

colon and to document the response to therapy. However, exact data about the accuracy of the Doppler sonography of splanchnic arteries in assessing disease activity are still lacking so far and, therefore, its use in routine clinical practice is still very limited.

3.5 Differential Diagnosis

The site and degree of bowel wall thickness and other features of the bowel wall may be helpful in differentiating between ulcerative colitis and Crohn's disease (Table 3.2), even if there are no specific ultrasonographic features of the intestinal walls that can be employed usefully in the differential diagnosis between ulcerative colitis and Crohn's disease. However, it has been reported that the sonographic features of the colonic wall may be useful to discriminate between ulcerative colitis and Crohn's disease in approximately 80 % of cases [29–31].

The ultrasonographic differential diagnosis between ulcerative colitis and acute inflammatory conditions such as infectious colitis, diverticular sigmoiditis and ischaemic lesions may be

Table 3.2 Main ultrasonographic features in differential diagnosis between ulcerative colitis and Crohn's disease

	Ulcerative colitis	Crohn's disease
Bowel wall		
Thickness	4–7 mm	5–14 mm
Echopattern	Variable	Variable
Vascularity	Variable	Variable
Contour	Well defined	Variable
Stiffness	Absent	Often present
Austra coli	Absent	Absent
Peristalsis		Often weak or absent
Location and extension		
Site	Recto-sigmoid and colon	Ileum (70 %), Colon (60)
Bowel involvement	Continuous	Often divided in segments
Extra-intestinal alterations		
Mesenteric hypertrophy	Uncommon	Common
Enlarged lymph nodes	Uncommon	Common
Fistulae and abscesses	Rare	Common

difficult. Infectious colitis shows a similar echopattern to that of ulcerative colitis, although infectious colitis is more frequently localized in the right colon and is more strongly associated with enlarged lymph nodes. Diverticular sigmoiditis differs from ulcerative colitis because the thickening is frequently segmental and eccentric, with diverticula on the outer border of the colon. Ischaemic colitis may be very difficult to differentiate from ulcerative colitis since the bowel wall thickening and echopattern may vary depending on the extent of devascularization and type of vascular obstruction. In this context, the study of splanchnic circulation may be useful.

References

1. Rompel O, Huelsse B, Bodenschatz K, Reutter G, Darge K (2006) Harmonic US imaging of appendicitis in children. Pediatr Radiol 36:1257–1264
2. Bluth EI, Merrit CR, Sullivan MA (1979) Ultrasonic evaluation of the stomach, small bowel and colon. Radiology 133:677–680
3. Worlicek H, Lutz H, Heyder N, Matek W (1987) Ultrasound findings in Crohn's disease and ulcerative colitis: a prospective study. J Clin Ultrasound 15:153–163
4. Maconi G, Sampietro GM, Ardizzone S et al (2004) US detection of toxic megacolon in inflammatory bowel diseases. Dig Dis Sci 49:138–142
5. Limberg B, Osswald B (1994) Diagnosis and differential diagnosis of ulcerative colitis and Crohn's disease by hydrocolonic sonography. Am J Gastroenterol 89:1051–1057
6. Pascu M, Roznowski AB, Muller HP, Adler A, Wiedenmann B, Dignass AU (2004) Clinical relevance of transabdominal ultrasonography and magnetic resonance imaging in patients with inflammatory bowel disease of the terminal ileum and large bowel. Inflamm Bowel Dis 10:373–382
7. Hollerbach S, Geissler A, Schiegl H et al (1998) The accuracy of abdominal ultrasound in the assessment of bowel disorders. Scand J Gastroenterol 33:1201–1208
8. Schwerk WB, Beckh K, Raith M (1992) A prospective evaluation of high resolution sonography in the diagnosis of inflammatory bowel diasease. Eur J Gastroenterol Hepatol 4:173–182
9. Worlicek H, Lutz H, Heyder N, Matek W (1987) Ultrasound findings in Crohn's disease and ulcerative colitis: a prospective study. J Clin Ultrasound 15:153–163
10. Hata J, Haruma K, Yamanaka H et al (1994) US evaluation of the bowel wall in inflammatory bowel disease: comparison of in vivo and in vitro studies. Abdom Imaging 19:395–399
11. Parente F, Greco S, Molteni M et al (2003) Role of early ultrasound in detecting inflammatory intestinal disorders and identifying their anatomical location within the bowel. Aliment Pharmacol Ther 18:1009–1016
12. Astegiano M, Bresso F, Cammarota T et al (2001) Abdominal pain and bowel dysfunction: diagnostic role of intestinal ultrasound. Eur J Gastroenterol Hepatol 13:927–931
13. Sonnenberg A, Erckenbrecht J, Peter P, Niederau C (1982) Detection of Crohn's disease by ultrasound. Gastroenterology 83:430–434
14. Arienti V, Campieri M, Boriani L et al (1996) Management of severe ulcerative colitis with the help of high resolution ultrasonography. Am J Gastroenterol 91:2163–2169
15. Maconi G, Ardizzone S, Parente F, Bianchi Porro G (1999) Ultrasonography in the evaluation of extension, activity, and follow-up of ulcerative colitis. Scand J Gastroenterol 34:1103–1107
16. Ruess L, Blask AR, Bulas DI (2000) Inflammatory bowel disease in children and young adults: correlation of sonographic and clinical parameters during treatment. AJR Am J Roentgenol 175:79–84
17. Bru C, Sans M, Defelitto MM et al (2001) Hydrocolonic sonography for evaluating inflammatory bowel disease. AJR Am J Roentgenol 177:99–105
18. Haber HP, Busch A, Ziebach R, Dette S, Ruck P, Stern M (2002) Ultrasonographic findings correspond to clinical, endoscopic, and histologic findings in inflammatory bowel disease and other enterocolitides. J Ultrasound Med 21:375–382
19. Antonelli E, Giuliano V, Casella G et al (2011) Ultrasonographic assessment of colonic wall in moderate-severe ulcerative colitis: comparison with endoscopic findings. Dig Liver Dis 43:703–706
20. Heyne R, Rickes S, Bock P, Schreiber S, Wermke W, Lochs H (2002) Non-invasive evaluation of activity in inflammatory bowel disease by power Doppler sonography. Z Gastroenterol 40:171–175
21. Parente F, Molteni M, Marino B et al (2010) Are colonoscopy and bowel ultrasound useful for assessing response to short-term therapy and predicting disease outcome of moderate-to-severe forms of ulcerative colitis? A prospective study. Am J Gastroenterol 105:1150–1157
22. Yoshida A, Kobayashi K, Ueno F et al (2011) Possible role of early transabdominal ultrasound in patients undergoing cytapheresis for active ulcerative colitis. Intern Med 50:11–15
23. Kalantzis N, Rouvella P, Tarazis S et al (2002) Doppler US of superior mesenteric artery in the assessment of ulcerative colitis: a prospective study. Hepatogastroenterology 49:168–171

24. Sigirci A, Baysal T, Kutlu R, Aladag M, Sarac K, Harputluoglu H (2001) Doppler sonography of the inferior and superior mesenteric arteries in ulcerative colitis. J Clin Ultrasound 29:130–139

25. Ludwig D, Wiener S, Bruning A et al (1999) Mesenteric blood flow is related to disease activity and risk of relapse in ulcerative colitis: a prospective follow up study. Gut 45:546–552

26. Mirk P, Palazzoni G, Gimondo P (1999) Doppler sonography of hemodynamic changes of the inferior mesenteric artery in inflammatory bowel disease: preliminary data. AJR Am J Roentgenol 173:381–387

27. Maconi G, Imbesi V, Bianchi Porro G (1996) Doppler ultrasound measurement of intestinal blood flow in inflammatory bowel disease. Scand J Gastroenterol 31:590–593

28. Bolondi L, Gaiani S, Brignola C et al (1992) Changes in splanchnic hemodynamics in inflammatory bowel disease. Non-invasive assessment by Doppler ultrasound flowmetry. Scand J Gastroenterol 27:501–507

29. Pera A, Cammarota T, Comino E et al (1988) Ultrasonography in the detection of Crohn's disease and in the differential diagnosis of inflammatory bowel disease. Digestion 41:180–184

30. Limberg B (1989) Diagnosis of acute ulcerative colitis and colonic Crohn's disease by colonic sonography. J Clin Ultrasound 17:25–31

31. Limberg B, Osswald B (1994) Diagnosis and differential diagnosis of ulcerative colitis and Croh's disease by hydrocolonic sonography. Am J Gastroenterol 89:1051–1057

Water Enema Multidetector CT Colonography: Technique, Role and Imaging Findings in Ulcerative Colitis

4

Alba H. Norsa and Massimo Tonolini

4.1 Introduction

Although optical colonoscopy (OC) remains the gold standard to investigate inflammatory and neoplastic colorectal disorders, after the introduction of multidetector scanners CT colonography (CTC) using air or carbon dioxide (CO_2) for colonic distension has become an established alternative technique, with a high sensitivity for detection of benign and malignant tumours. The main advantages of CTC include good patient acceptance and tolerability compared to OC, feasibility in patients with impossible or incomplete endoscopy and a limited radiation dose with acquisition protocols used for screening purposes. Furthermore, contrast-enhanced CTC with full radiation dose is an established staging modality in patients with known or suspected colorectal carcinoma. However, CTC has some intrinsic drawbacks, including the need of specific equipment for CO_2 insufflation, a double acquisition in supine and prone positions and time-consuming image analysis and interpretation by experienced radiologists [1–4].

Recently, some authors investigated CTC in the assessment of large bowel abnormalities in patients with idiopathic inflammatory bowel diseases (IBD), such as mural thickening, lumen narrowing, loss of haustration and pseudopolyps. The limited published experiences yielded conflicting results, with unsatisfactory visualization of mucosal abnormalities, and assessment of mural thickening hampered by wall compression from luminal air overdistension. Furthermore, in this population air insufflation should be performed carefully because the inflamed, more fragile intestinal wall poses a greater risk of colonic perforation [5–7].

As from the European Crohn's and colitis organization (ECCO) guidelines and the recent ECCO–European society of gastrointestinal and abdominal radiology (ESGAR) consensus guidelines, currently, the limited available data do not demonstrate an adequate diagnostic value of CT or CTC for assessing the disease extent and activity in UC [8–10].

According to the same joint consensus [8], imaging the large bowel in IBD requires luminal distension and intravenous contrast administration, and should be performed using a multidetector scanner to cover the entire abdomen and pelvis in a single breath-hold, with thin detector collimation to provide high-quality multiplanar reformations. In order to further minimize motion and peristaltic artefacts, the addition of pharmacological hypotonisation should prove beneficial.

A. H. Norsa (✉)
Radiology, "Sant'Ambrogio" Clinical Institute, Via Faravelli 16, 20149 Milan, Italy
e-mail: alba.norsa@gmail.com

M. Tonolini
Radiology Department, "Luigi Sacco" University Hospital, Via G.B. Grassi 74, 20157 Milan, Italy
e-mail: mtonolini@sirm.org

M. Tonolini (ed.), *Imaging of Ulcerative Colitis*,
DOI: 10.1007/978-88-470-5409-7_4, © Springer-Verlag Italia 2014

Water enema multidetector CT (WE-MDCT) couples retrograde colonic distension using water with mural enhancement by intravenous contrast medium, provides excellent visualization of the enhanced colonic wall and good contrast between the wall itself, the hypodense lumen and the pericolonic fat. Currently, WE-MDCT is increasingly proposed as the most accurate imaging technique in patients with suspected or proven colorectal neoplasms [11–14] and to diagnose bowel endometriosis [15, 16]. Advantages of WE-MDCT over air CTC include a simpler acquisition in the supine position only, and a short learning curve without need for complex post-processing. WE-MDCT provides a panoramic multiplanar visualization of intestinal abnormalities, associated extramural findings and complications, with sub-millimeter spatial resolution reproducing the classical orientation of double-contrast barium enema which is familiar to most surgeons [4].

Optimally tolerated, WE-MDCT provides a very accurate evaluation of wall thickness and enhancement in normal and pathologic conditions, and detailed visualization of associated perivisceral and extraintestinal abnormalities. Therefore, WE-MDCT represents an appealing modality to investigate also chronic IBD of the large bowel, particularly when endoscopy is incomplete, or with possible complications involving the perivisceral planes or adjacent organs [4, 7, 17, 18].

4.2 Water Enema Multidetector CT Technique and Interpretation

4.2.1 Bowel Preparation and Contraindications

At our Department, prior to elective WE-MDCT patients receive a standard oral bowel preparation consisting in a laxative iso-osmolar non-absorbable solution of polyethylene glycol powder such as 4–6 doses of Isocolan (Bracco, Milan-Italy) each dissolved in 500 ml water or 3–4 doses of SELG-ESSE 1000 (Promefarm, Milan-Italy) each dissolved in 1 l of water the day before the examination, in association with a low-residue diet for 3 days. Patients then fast for 12 h after a liquid dinner the evening before the scheduled examination [4, 15, 16].

Although preliminary bowel cleansing should be obtained, unless contraindicated by emergency conditions or poor performance status, as discussed in Chap. 6 this book dealing with acute UC manifestations, we have performed WE-MDCT with no or limited bowel preparation such as with laxative (sennosides) capsules plus magnesium citrate solution, in some patients with acute intestinal symptoms to stage UC, confirm activity and obviate a risky endoscopy. However, we do not perform nor recommend WE-MDCT without bowel preparation when toxic megacolon, free perforation and acute peritonitis are clinically suspected or radiographically detected. In patients with clinical and/or radiographic diagnosis of large bowel obstruction, which is caused by colorectal carcinoma (CRC) in almost 60 % of cases, retrograde colonic distension is unnecessary because standard contrast-enhanced MDCT reliably evaluates the site and underlying cause of obstruction thanks to the intrinsic contrast provided by the upstream dilatation with endoluminal fluid [4].

4.2.2 Patient Preparation

In the CT suite, patient preparation is performed by experienced radiology nurses, with gentle insertion of a lubricated enema tube into the rectum with the patient lying on the CT scanner table in the left lateral decubitus position. The tube is then connected to a bag that contains 2 l of warm tap water, and retrograde colonic distension is obtained through gravity during 3–5 min. Afterward, the patient is instructed to turn on his right side to improve water distribution, and is then positioned supine for CT acquisition. Alternatively, incontinent patients may have enema performed by use of an inflatable balloon tip [4].

Unless contraindicated, we routinely administer pharmacological hypotonisation with 20 mg hyoscine butylbromide (Buscopan, Boehringer

Ingelheim, Florence, Italy) intravenously injected prior to water enema. Hypotonization improves patient comfort, enhances colonic wall elasticity resulting in easier distension and reduces peristalsis and motion artefacts. Thus, better assessment of the true mural thickness is achieved, along with the reduction of visceral spasms which could be confused with stenosis [4].

4.2.3   Exam Acquisition Protocol and Safety

Volumetric CT acquisition of the abdomen and pelvis during a single breath-hold is then performed during intravenous injection of 110–130 ml of nonionic iodinated contrast medium (such as 350 mgI/mL iomeprol or 370 mgI/mL iopromide) using an automated power injection at a 2.5 ml/s flow rate, with a 75 s scan delay. Acquisition parameters on a 64-slice CT scanner include 120 kV, 300 mAs, 0.891 pitch, 0.75 s rotation time and 64 × 0.625 mm collimation. The estimated radiation dose erogated during WE-MDCT acquisition using this protocol is usually in the range 12–14 mGy [4].

Then, water enema is drained before the patient leaves the CT suite. The total examination time lasts for about 10 min. In agreement with other Authors, in our experience preliminary preparation and examination are well tolerated by the majority of patients, and we have not observed any adverse effects or complications related to the procedure [4, 14].

4.2.4   Exam Interpretation and Pitfalls

WE-MDCT is a reproducible technique that does not need complex post processing or 3D interpretation, therefore a very short learning curve is to be expected in radiologists who are familiar with abdominal studies [14]. Images are routinely reconstructed along axial, coronal and sagittal planes; however, the attending radiologist usually reviews the study on a dedicated workstation with the possibility to save arbitrary reconstruction images focused on the key

findings, including oblique or curved-planar reformations [4].

In WE-MDCT, optimal contrast is observed between the well-distended lumen with water density, the enhanced colonic wall and the normal fat-density pericolonic planes (Fig. 4.1). The mural thickness should be measured in non-dependent, well-distended portions and should not exceed 2–3 mm. During exam interpretation, radiologists should carefully search for non-distensible segments along the large bowel with or without prestenotic dilatations (diameter over 5 cm), signs of mural thickening, hyperenhancement and/or stratification, endoluminal projections and diverticular outpouchings. Perivisceral fat changes such as increased density, hypervascularization, adipose proliferation or adenopathies should be sought for. Furthermore, WE-MDCT allows comprehensive imaging of associated or incidental abnormalities involving the abdominal organs, lymph nodes, peritoneum, mesentery, retroperitoneum, lumbar and pelvic skeleton [4].

Potential pitfalls of the technique are mostly represented by non-distended bowel segments, and by the presence of fecal residues, which is the rule when bowel preparation is limited or avoided. Whereas other authors have reported a 95 % sensitivity and specificity for the detection of CRC in unclean bowel, in our experience endoluminal stools usually do not hamper a correct assessment of the colonic wall thickness and enhancement pattern, but sub-centimeter polyps and fine mural details characteristic of UC may be obscured [4, 11, 14].

4.3   Water Enema Multidetector CT in Ulcerative Colitis

4.3.1   Mural WE-MDCT Findings

Pathologically, UC is characterized by extensive mucosal ulceration and diffuse non-granulomatous inflammation that usually commences in the rectum and extends proximally in a continuous, confluent and concentric manner to affect a variable entity of the large bowel.

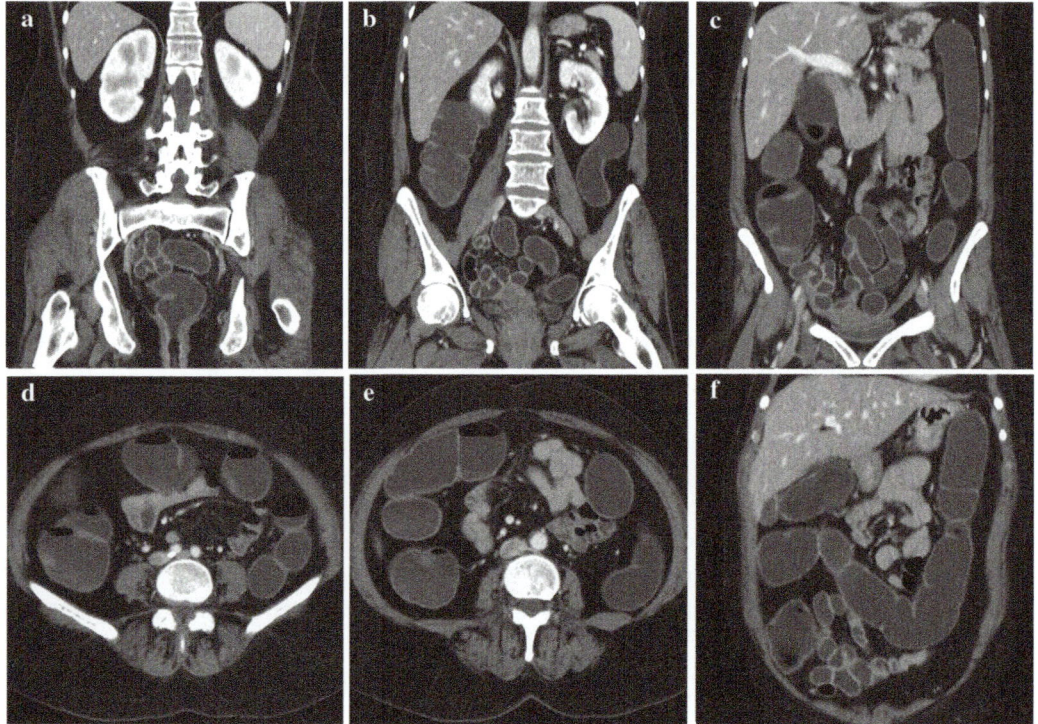

Fig. 4.1 Normal water enema multidetector CT (WE-MDCT) examination in a 55-year-old woman with unspecific abdominal complaints, requested to investigate clinical suspicion of diverticulitis. Image review along coronal and axial planes allows assessing all well-distended segments of the large bowel, with optimal contrast between the perivisceral fat, thin enhanced colonic wall and hypodense lumen. No non-distended segments, mural thickening or intraluminal vegetations are observed. Faecal residues are absent following standard bowel preparation. Note rectal tube in (**a**)

Historically, CT had a limited role in imaging patients with UC, because of its low sensitivity for endoscopically detected early disease changes [7, 19].

However, despite being primarily a mucosal disease, UC is commonly characterized by mural colon thickening. Therefore, with its intrinsic optimal spatial resolution, tissue contrast, luminal and mural distension, WE-MDCT may usefully complement OC to assess the colonic wall in its full-thickness, as well as mesenteric and extraintestinal changes. Early superficial and flat mucosal changes observed at OC, such as granulation due to oedema, hyperemia and increased mucin secretion, remain below the high resolution power of MDCT [7, 18].

In patients with UC, WE-MDCT allows an easy identification of the transition between the involved large bowel which is not completely distended despite pharmacological hypotonisation, and the upstream spared segments that usually appear well distended with recognizable haustral folds. Most usually, UC changes show a continuous distribution from the rectum (which is spared in 4 % of cases only) to the left-sided or the entire colon (Figs. 4.2, 4.3 and 4.4). In UC, colon wall thickening is usually of moderate entity (6−9 mm), circumferential and symmetric in the majority of cases. In the only series that investigated the role of MDCT in UC, wall thickening was positively associated with endoscopic, clinical and histopathological severity [4, 18]

Whereas WE-MDCT findings observed in active UC phases are discussed in Chap. 6 dealing with acute UC manifestations of this book, with disease progression mucosal ulceration and denudation leading to the formation of inflammatory pseudopolyps, which can be

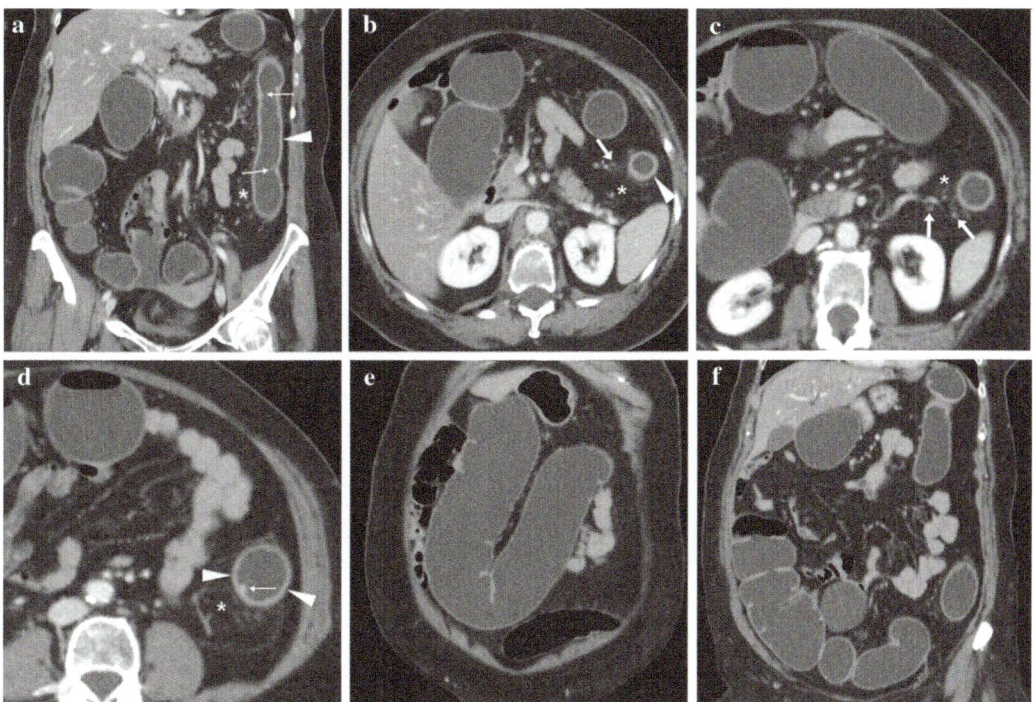

Fig. 4.2 63-year-old female with ulcerative colitis. Elective WE-MDCT shows moderate, uniform mural thickening throughout the descending colon (*arrowheads*) with tiny endoluminal projections corresponding to endoscopic finding of pseudopolyps (*thin arrows*). The proliferating pericolonic fat shows increased density and vascularity (*) with some tiny lymph nodes (*arrows*). The upstream transverse and *right* colon is well distended with preserved haustra (Reprinted from Open Access Ref. [4])

visualized at WE-MDCT as tiny solid endoluminal projections (Figs. 4.2, 4.3 and 4.4). In subacute and chronic phases of UC, the characteristic marked hypertrophy of the muscularis mucosa and transmural fibrosis produces diffuse, uniform mural thickening, reduced distension and shortening of the involved colon, segmental or diffuse luminal narrowing (Figs. 4.2, 4.3 and 4.4) [4, 7, 18, 19].

4.3.2   Proposed Indications for WE-MDCT in Ulcerative Colitis

According to the above-cited current clinical guidelines, indications for CT in UC should be limited to cases of impossible or incomplete OC (Figs. 4.3, 4.4), and impassable stenosis. Due to the substantial CRC risk, the endoscopic detection of a colonic stricture in UC warrants further imaging investigation with WE-MDCT, to assess both its features and the upstream colon (Fig. 4.4) [4, 8].

Furthermore, in our experience selected patients with UC and incomplete endoscopy may benefit from WE-MDCT to determine the longitudinal disease extent. In fact, the distribution of UC according to the Montreal criteria as proctitis, left-sided (distal to the splenic flexure) or extensive colitis (including pancolitis) influences patient management (particularly the choice of drug delivery system), dictates CRC risk and therefore the start and frequency of periodic surveillance [4, 9, 10, 20].

Finally, WE-MDCT may be helpful when discrepancy exists between clinical and endoscopic findings, such as in suspected UC with a discontinuous endoscopic appearance of colonic inflammation, and in patients with unclear IBD classification between UC and CD [4, 8].

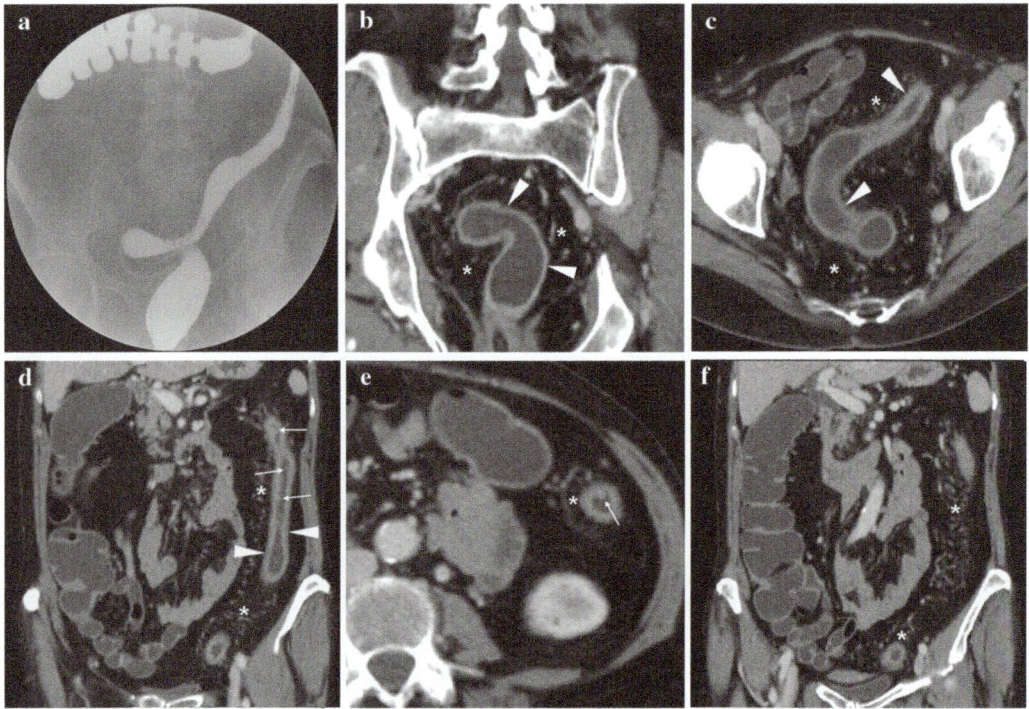

Fig. 4.3 65-year-old female with ulcerative colitis, initially investigated with water-soluble contrast enema shows "water-pipe" appearance of shortened, narrow *left* colon with advanced haustral loss (**a**). After medical treatment, elective WE-MDCT was performed because of incomplete colonoscopy. Discrete, circumferential mural thickening is observed from the rectum to the splenic flexure (*arrowheads*), corresponding to endoscopic severe disease, with confirmation of several millimetric pseudopolyps (*thin arrows*) throughout the descending tract. Markedly increased vascularity is seen in the proliferating perirectal and pericolonic fat planes (***). Most of the transverse and *right* colon appear to be spared (Reprinted from Open Access Ref. [4])

4.3.3 Perivisceral WE-MDCT Findings

Additional extraintestinal changes observed in UC include proliferation of pericolonic fat with hyperemia and vascular engorgement, a slightly increased attenuation (10−20 HU) compared to normal abdominal fat due to oedema and inflammation, often containing nodular densities corresponding to enlarged lymph nodes (Figs. 4.2, 4.3 and 4.4). These changes are more consistently identifiable and highly suggestive of UC in the perirectal area, resulting in pathologic (over 15 mm) widening of the presacral space, which is measured from the posterior rectal wall to the anterior cortex of the sacrum [4, 7, 18].

In chronic stages of UC, the colon submucosa undergoes widening and adipose infiltration, resulting in the "fat halo sign" mural stratification with a fat-density intermediate ring separating the bowel mucosa from the outer soft-tissue muscularis propria and serosa, a finding that is seen by far more commonly in UC (61 %) than in CD (8 % of cases) [4, 21–23].

4.3.4 Colorectal Cancer in Ulcerative Colitis

Although patients with UC usually undergo periodic OC, due to the substantial risk of CRC WE-MDCT studies in UC, patients should be carefully scrutinized to identify features that suggest an underlying malignancy, particularly in patients with failed endoscopic surveillance or incomplete endoscopy. As discussed in Chap. 10 of this book, a soft-tissue mass, or a mural thickening which is greater than 1.5 cm,

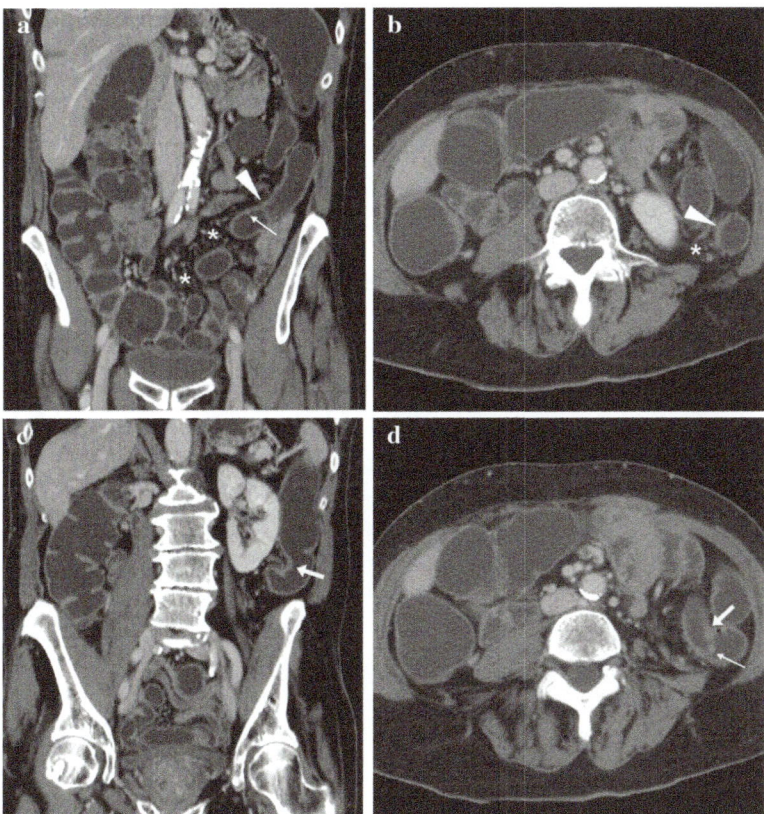

Fig. 4.4 63-year-old male with ulcerative colonoscopy and endoscopy limited to 45 cm from the anal verge because of non-distensible colon with diffuse mucosal changes and pseudopolyps. Elective WE-MDCT shows moderate mural thickening throughout the rectosigmoid and descending tract consistent with *left*-sided colitis (*arrowheads*) and associated pericolonic fat changes (*). In the proximal descending colon, a focal substenosis with asymmetric mural thickening (*arrows*) and pseudopolyps (*thin arrow*) is detected, prompting endoscopic and bioptic re-evaluation, that allowed to exclude carcinoma and dysplasia. Fair distension of the transverse and *right* colon with preserved mural thickness and haustra (Reprinted from Open Access Ref. [4])

asymmetric and/or with homogeneous solid attenuation and focal loss of mural stratification should be promptly reported as suspicious and needing biopsy. In our opinion, the use of WE-MDCT should probably improve the limited accuracy reported for detection of CRC in the setting of IBD [4, 7, 9, 10, 24].

4.3.5   Differentiation Versus Crohn's Disease and Indeterminate Colitis

Compared to UC, colonic Crohn's disease (CD) mural thickening is usually segmental and discontinuous, with affected regions alternating with spared "skip" tracts, and of a greater entity (11−13 mm vs. 7−8 mm in UC). The characteristic involvement of the distal ileum may be detected by WE-MDCT, allowing differentiation from UC. The distribution of perivisceral fat changes also differs, involving the right-sided mesentery around the terminal ileum and ileocecal valve in CD, whereas the presacral space is characteristically involved in UC. Intense contrast enhancement of the inflamed mucosa and "target" appearance is seen during active CD phases, whereas long-standing disease develops transmural fibrosis resulting in loss of mural stratification and lesser, homogeneous mural enhancement which may resemble UC.

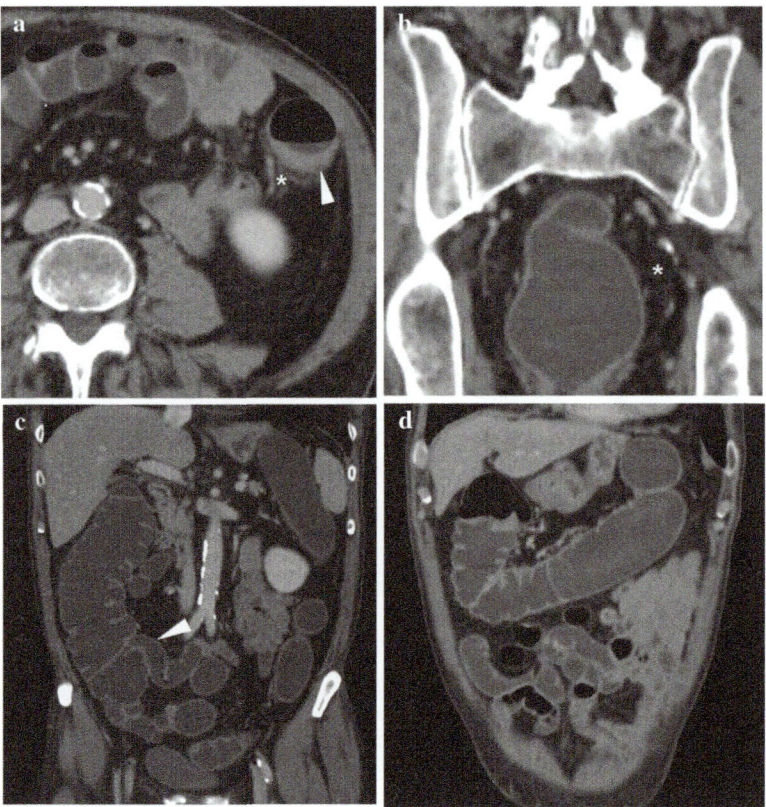

Fig. 4.5 A 69-year-old male with clinical, endoscopic and bioptic diagnosis of indeterminate colitis. WE-MDCT requested to further characterize the disease yielded good distension of the large bowel, with perirectal and pericolonic fat changes (*) and moderate asymmetric mural thickening of the descending colon (*arrowhead*), findings closely resembling those of a *left-*sided ulcerative colitis. Suspicion of Crohn's disease is excluded by the normal appearance of the well-distended terminal ileum (*arrowhead* in **c**) (Partially reprinted from Open Access Ref. [4])

Similarly to UC, early and superficial CD changes such as enlarged lymphoid follicles and aphthoid ulcers limited to the mucosa cannot be resolved by MDCT [19, 21, 22].

Currently, the term indeterminate colitis is adopted by pathologists when a histological specimen shows overlapping features between CD and UC. Clinically, "colitis yet to be classified" should be adopted for the minority (up to 6 %) of patients where a definitive distinction between UC and CD cannot be made on the basis of history, endoscopy, histopathology and appropriate radiologic studies [10]. In these patients, WE-MDCT may be performed as a complement to OC, to investigate disease distribution and features of mural and

extraintestinal changes, and may, to some degree, contribute to the differential diagnosis between CD and UC (Fig. 4.5) [7].

4.3.6 Drawbacks of Water Enema Multidetector CT: The Radiation Issue

As clearly stated in the ECCO-ESGAR consensus guidelines, cross-sectional imaging currently plays a pivotal role in the diagnosis and management of patients with IBD. However, increasing use of MDCT causes concern about the potential malignancy risk associated to ionizing radiation. Radiation exposure is by far the key limitation of MDCT, particularly in patients with IBD who require frequent examinations throughout their lifelong course. The risk of radiation-induced cancer is increased by both MDCT radiation burden and earlier age of exposure [8].

A few years ago, a retrospective study assessed the cumulative ionizing radiation exposure expressed in milli-Sieverts (mSv) from abdominal imaging studies in an IBD cohort over a 5-year time span, and disclosed that 7 % of CD patients were exposed to high levels of radiation (>50 mSv), in contrast to no patient with UC [25]. More recently, a meta-analysis including 1,704 patients in six studies calculated the proportion of patients receiving a potentially harmful ≥ 50 mSv dose, which globally approximates one out of ten (8.8 %) IBD patients, with a significant difference between CD and UC (11.1 % vs. 2 % prevalence, respectively), and strong correlation with corticosteroid use and IBD surgery [26].

In conclusion, considering the awareness of the radiation exposure risks and the increasing role of MDCT in the assessment of IBD patients in elective and urgent conditions, efforts should be made to minimize exposure from MDCT by limiting the number of studies, by employing alternative imaging modalities such as ultrasound (with the drawback of poor panoramicity) and MRI (which has unfortunately a limited spatial resolution compared to WE-MDCT) and by adopting low-dose MDCT acquisition protocols [25].

References

1. Pickhardt PJ, Wise SM, Kim DH (2010) Positive predictive value for polyps detected at screening CT colonography. Eur Radiol 20:1651–1656
2. Pickhardt PJ, Hassan C, Halligan S et al (2011) Colorectal cancer: CT colonography and colonoscopy for detection–systematic review and meta-analysis. Radiology 259:393–405
3. Neri E, Halligan S, Hellstrom M et al (2012) The second ESGAR consensus statement on CT colonography. Eur Radiol 23:720–729
4. Norsa AH, Tonolini M, Ippolito S et al (2013) Water enema multidetector CT technique and imaging of diverticulitis and chronic inflammatory bowel diseases. Insights Imaging 4:309–20
5. Tarjan Z, Zagoni T, Gyorke T et al (2000) Spiral CT colonography in inflammatory bowel disease. Eur J Radiol 35:193–198
6. Carrascosa P, Castiglioni R, Capunay C et al (2007) CT colonoscopy in inflammatory bowel disease. Abdom Imaging 32:596–601
7. Regge D, Neri E, Turini F et al (2009) Role of CT colonography in inflammatory bowel disease. Eur J Radiol 69:404–408
8. Panes J, Bouhnik Y, Reinisch W et al (2013) Imaging techniques for assessment of inflammatory bowel disease: joint ECCO and ESGAR evidence-based consensus guidelines. J Crohns Colitis 7:556–85
9. Biancone L, Michetti P, Travis S et al (2008) European evidence-based Consensus on the management of ulcerative colitis: special situations. J Crohns Colitis 2:63–92
10. Stange EF, Travis SP, Vermeire S et al (2008) European evidence-based Consensus on the diagnosis and management of ulcerative colitis: definitions and diagnosis. J Crohns Colitis 2:1–23
11. Soyer P, Sirol M, Dray X et al (2012) Detection of colorectal tumors with water enema-multidetector row computed tomography. Abdom Imaging 37:1092–1100
12. Soyer P, Hamzi L, Sirol M et al (2012) Colon cancer: comprehensive evaluation with 64-section CT colonography using water enema as intraluminal contrast agent-a pictorial review. Clin Imaging 36:113–125
13. Ridereau-Zins C, Sibileau E, Pavageau AH et al (2011) Accuracy of water enema-MDCT in colon cancer staging: a prospective study. Cancer Imaging 11(A):S115
14. Ridereau-Zins C, Aube C, Luet D et al (2010) Assessment of water enema computed tomography: an effective imaging technique for the diagnosis of colon cancer: colon cancer: computed tomography using a water enema. Abdom Imaging 35:407–413
15. Biscaldi E, Ferrero S, Remorgida V et al (2007) Bowel endometriosis: CT-enteroclysis. Abdom Imaging 32:441–450
16. Biscaldi E, Ferrero S, Fulcheri E et al (2007) Multislice CT enteroclysis in the diagnosis of bowel endometriosis. Eur Radiol 17:211–219
17. Paparo F, Bacigalupo L, Garello I et al (2012) Crohn's disease: prevalence of intestinal and extraintestinal manifestations detected by computed tomography enterography with water enema. Abdom Imaging 37:326–337
18. Patel B, Mottola J, Sahni VA et al (2012) MDCT assessment of ulcerative colitis: radiologic analysis with clinical, endoscopic, and pathologic correlation. Abdom Imaging 37:61–69
19. Gore RM, Balthazar EJ, Ghahremani GG et al (1996) CT features of ulcerative colitis and Crohn's disease. AJR Am J Roentgenol 167:3–15

20. Zisman TL, Rubin DT (2008) Colorectal cancer and dysplasia in inflammatory bowel disease. World J Gastroenterol 14:2662–2669
21. Horton KM, Corl FM, Fishman EK (2000) CT evaluation of the colon: inflammatory disease. Radiographics 20:399–418
22. Thoeni RF, Cello JP (2006) CT imaging of colitis. Radiology 240:623–638
23. Ahualli J (2007) The fat halo sign. Radiology 242:945–946
24. Hristova L, Soyer P, Hoeffel C et al (2012) Colorectal cancer in inflammatory bowel diseases: CT features with pathological correlation. Abdom Imaging 38:421–35
25. Kroeker KI, Lam S, Birchall I et al (2011) Patients with IBD are exposed to high levels of ionizing radiation through CT scan diagnostic imaging: a five-year study. J Clin Gastroenterol 45:34–39
26. Chatu S, Subramanian V, Pollok RC (2012) Meta-analysis: diagnostic medical radiation exposure in inflammatory bowel disease. Aliment Pharmacol Ther 35:529–539

Magnetic Resonance Imaging of Ulcerative Colitis

5

Francesca Maccioni and Fabrizio Mazzamurro

5.1 Introduction

Magnetic resonance imaging (MRI) is an excellent modality to investigate the entire bowel and can play an important role in the overall evaluation of IBD (Inflammatory Bowel Disease), definitely an important field of interest for gastrointestinal radiologists [1]. The intrinsic properties of MRI, such as high contrast resolution, availability of multiple imaging parameters, high sensitivity for inflammation of T2-weighted and T1-weighted gadolinium-enhanced sequences, make it a valuable diagnostic tool for IBD. Crohn's disease (CD) and ulcerative colitis (UC) are the two major chronic inflammatory bowel diseases, both widely diffused in western countries. Although CD and UC share a common unknown origin and a chronic relapsing/remitting course that lasts for the patient's lifetime, they show different macroscopic and microscopic features. UC is a chronic, idiopathic, inflammatory disease that involves almost exclusively the rectal and colonic mucosa, with a continuous spreading and predictable course and localization, while CD affects the small and large bowel in a discontinuous and unpredictable way.

Moreover, while CD is characterized by a transmural inflammation which involves all wall layers, UC is rather characterized by mural inflammation confined to the mucosal and submucosal layers only, with aphthoid ulcers, mucosal edema, lymphocyte infiltration and disruption of mucosal elements, without extramural involvement [2, 3].

Due to these relevant differences, CD and UC have a different clinical and diagnostic management. The final diagnosis of CD, usually more difficult to achieve, is based on the clinical evaluation and on the results of several instrumental examinations, including endoscopy (ES), radiology, MRI or other cross-sectional imaging modalities and histopathology [4]. Conversely, the endoscopic evaluation alone is usually sufficient to assess the extent and severity of UC, since its inflammatory process involves the colon only, sparing the small bowel [3]. Biopsy specimens can usually detect most of the pathologic features of UC, since the inflammatory process does not extend beyond the submucosa layer, differently from CD where inflammation involves all wall layers.

In UC, however, endoscopy may be contraindicated in the acute phases of the disease due to the high risk of perforation, or it can be incomplete for technical reasons or refused by the patient, in up to 30 % of cases [5]. Late complications of UC, particularly tight strictures, can partially or completely prevent the

F. Maccioni (✉) · F. Mazzamurro
Department of Radiological Sciences, Oncology and Pathology, University of Rome "Sapienza", Viale Regina Elena 324, 00161 Rome, Italy
e-mail: Francesca.maccioni@uniroma1.it

F. Mazzamurro
e-mail: fmazzamurro@libero.it

M. Tonolini (ed.), *Imaging of Ulcerative Colitis*,
DOI: 10.1007/978-88-470-5409-7_5, © Springer-Verlag Italia 2014

passage of an endoscope. In all these cases MRI may play a crucial role in the evaluation and characterization of UC [3–5].

5.2 Technique

For evaluation of the bowel, MRI should be performed with highly performing magnets and phased array coils [6–10].

5.2.1 Intestinal Preparation and Contrast Agents

To avoid signal inhomogeneities related to residual stools, patients should undergo satisfactory colon cleaning by drinking nearly 2–3 litres of iso-osmolar water solution (e.g. polyethylene glycol solution), approximately 18–12 h before the examination, with the exception of those with severe diarrhoea. In the evaluation of IBD, the oral administration of contrast agents is recommended, in order to achieve a homogenous signal at the level of both small and large bowel loops. Intestinal contrast agents may produce either a negative or a positive lumen effect, according to different sequences.

Super paramagnetic intestinal contrast agents (suspension of iron oxide particles) produce a negative effect both on T1- or T2-weighted imaging [6–10], improving the evidence of wall gadolinium enhancement on T1-weighted images and clearly displaying the bowel wall oedema on T2-weighted ones (Table 5.1). The transit of this contrast agent through the small bowel is rapid in patients with IBDs; an adequate opacification of the entire colon can be obtained 60−90 min after oral administration of 900−1,000 cc. They are usually used in adult patients, being less tolerated by children.

Retrograde air inflation may be useful to distend the colon, the air having a negative contrast effect, although it may be risky in case of severe colonic inflammation and less tolerated by patients.

Alternatively, biphasic contrast agents such as polyethylene glycol, may be used, producing a negative effect on T1-w and a positive effect on T2-w images.

Biphasic contrast agents are frequently used in IBD, being easily available and inexpensive [6–10] (Fig. 5.2). They are more effective on T1-weighted imaging and balanced imaging (True-FISP, FIESTA) rather than with T2-weighted imaging, due to inhomogeneous signal related to frequent flow-void artefacts.

Table 5.1 Technical parameters and suggested association of sequence/contrast agents

	T2 w HASTE	T2 w fat-suppressed HASTE	T2 w BLADE-TSE	True FISP	T1 w VIBE
Repetition time (ms)	1,000	1,000	3,880	3.5	6
Echo time (ms)	85	85	130	1,46	2.7/3
Section thickness (mm)	5–6	6	5–6	4	3/3.5
Slice/s	30/20 s	30/23 s	10/20 s	30/20 s	30/19 s
Slice gap (%)	10 %–0	10 %	10 %	15 %	3D
Matrix	256 × 182	256 × 182	356 × 256	256 × 182	256 × 159
FOV (mm$_2$): variable	350	350	350 × 350	350	350
Flip angle (°)	150–180	150–180	150	60	10
Slice orientation	Axial-corona	Axial	Axial-coronal	Axial-coronal	Axial-coronal
Gadolinium chelate iv	–	–	–	–	60 s delay
Negative superparamagnetic contrast agent	Yes	Yes	Yes	No	Yes
Biphasic contrast agent	Multiple artefacts	No	No	Yes	Yes

5.2.2 Sequences

MRI assessment of IBD should always include T1-weighted sequences after gadolinium injection for the excellent display of bowel wall inflammation. These sequences, available in 2D or 3D breath hold acquisition, with and without fat suppression, are labelled in different ways in different MR systems (FSPGR, VIBE, Thrive, etc.) and characterized by a short acquisition time (<1 s for slice). A 60 s delay after gadolinium injection is adequate to obtain a good assessment of the wall and mesenteric vascularity.

Suppression of the fat signal is mandatory for the evaluation of wall enhancement after gadolinium injection, although it may obscure evidence of mesenteric lymph nodes [7–9].

T2-weighted sequences are very sensitive in detecting inflammatory tissues, but only under adequate image conditions and with optimal and intestinal contrast, particularly in association with negative superparamagnetic contrast agents. Half-Fourier single-shot turbo spin-echo (HASTE) T2-weighted sequences are commonly used in the evaluation of the bowel, in breath hold or breath hold free acquisition, being

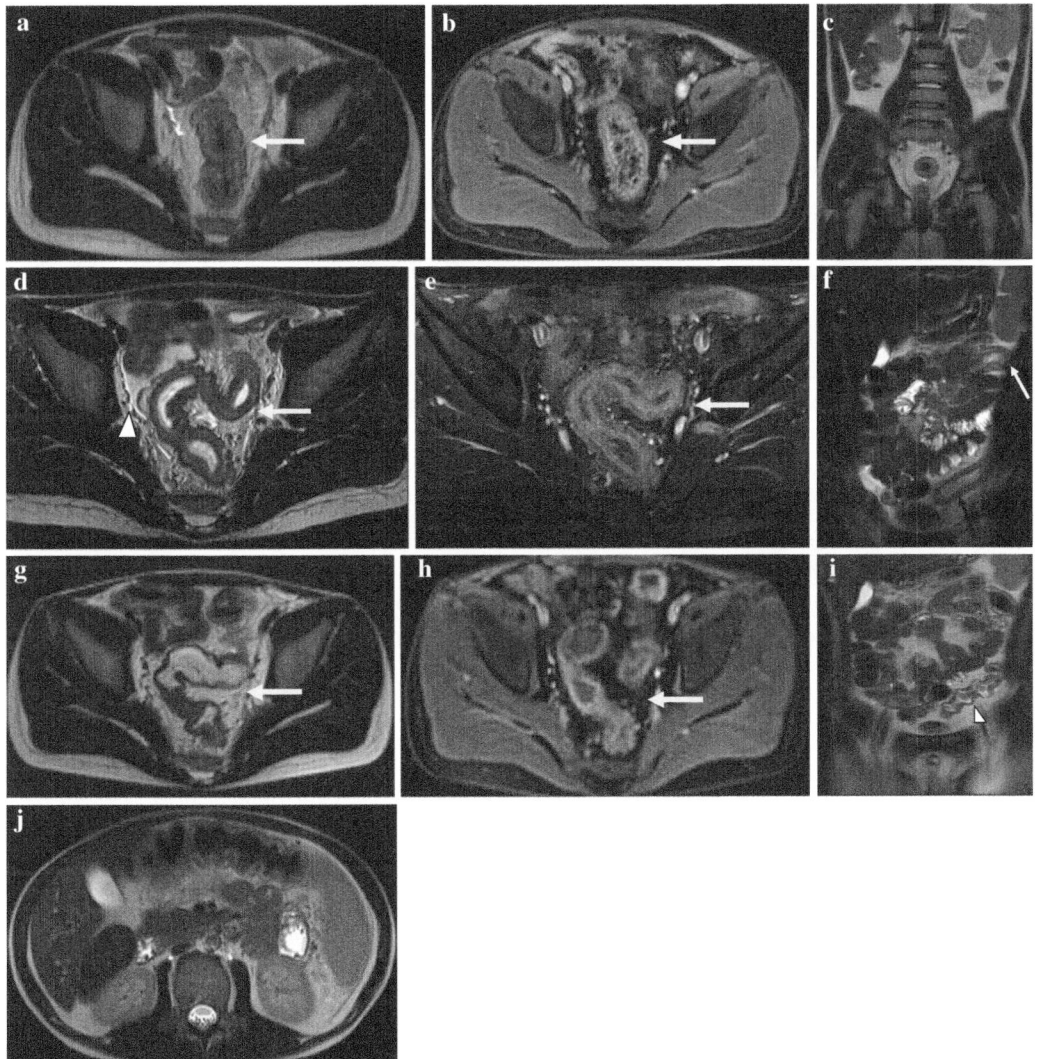

◀ **Fig. 5.1** 9-year-old boy, with severe bloody diarrhoea and weight loss, affected by UC as confirmed at endoscopy and histology. Three consecutive MRI studies were performed within a period of 14 months from the initial diagnosis, showing caudocranial progression of the colonic disease in spite of the pharmacological therapy. No oral contrast was administered due to low patient compliance. Starting with a prevalent severe involvement of the rectum and sigmoid colon, observed in the first examination, the disease progressed to a severe involvement of the *left* colon in the second examination and the transverse colon, in the third one. The patient was finally treated with total proctocolectomy and ileo-anal pouch. For a direct comparison, the axial images of the three different examinations are shown consequentially, as well as the coronal views. The first examination includes (**a**, **b** and **c**), the second, performed 10 months after the first one, includes (**d**, **e** and **f**) and the third examination, performed 3 months after the previous (**g**, **h**, **i** and **j**). Axial T2-weighted half-Fourier single-shot turbo spin-echo (**a**), axial T1-weighted gadolinium-enhanced images (**b**) and coronal T2-weighted half-Fourier single-shot turbo spin-echo

(**c**) of the first examination show diffuse wall thickening of the sigmoid colon and extensive Gd-enhancement, suggesting severe inflammation. Notice that the external wall profile is very regular even in very active disease, due to the prevalent inflammation of the inner wall layers (**a** *white arrow*). Axial images of the second examination (**d** and **e**) show only minimal reduction of wall thickness in the sigmoid colon, severe wall inflammation being still evident. Notice the minimal amount of perivisceral free fluid (*white arrow head*), suggesting acute disease. On the coronal image (**f**) a continuous inflammatory involvement from the proximal sigmoid colon up to the splenic flexure (**f** *white arrow*) is observed, with loss of the colonic haustra and tubular aspect of the bowel (**f** *black arrow*), due to severe wall oedema. In the third and last examination (**g**, **h**, **i** and **j**) there is a further reduction of wall thickness and a recovery of the austral folds (**i** *white arrow head*) in the *left* colon, due to reduced wall inflammation, as also confirmed at endoscopy. Unfortunately, the disease progressed and worsened in the transverse colon (**j**). Due to persistence of severe symptoms the patient underwent total colectomy.

characterized by a very short acquisition time (<1 slice/s). Having high intrinsic contrast and adequate spatial resolution (Figs. 5.1a, c, f, g, h, i, j, 5.3a, b), they are effective in detecting bowel wall and mesenteric inflammation, both with and without fatsuppression [9]. Balanced sequences (true-FISP Fiesta), T1 and T2-weighted images are valuable in association with a biphasic in contrast agents (Fig. 5.2a, b).

5.3 Assessment of Intestinal Disease and Perivisceral Manifestations

5.3.1 Intestinal Wall Characterization

The typical inflammatory process of UC, being confined to the mucosal and submucosal layers only, determines mild wall thickness with sparing of outer layers (muscularis propria and serosa). Colonic wall thickening is, in fact, usually lower in UC than in CD, with a mean value of 7 mm versus 13 mm, respectively, as reported in previous CT studies [4, 11–13]. At MRI, it can be detected both on T1- and T2-weighted images (Fig. 5.3). In very acute phases, however,

thickening of the colonic wall may exceed 10 mm, making it difficult to differentiate UC from CD (Fig. 5.1a, b).

The inner profile of the wall frequently shows a waved configuration both in UC and CD. The outer profile of the intestinal wall, instead, is sharper and smoother in UC than in CD, due to the intramural rather than transmural extent of the inflammatory process (Fig. 5.1). The outer contour of the colonic wall is smooth and regular in up to 95 % of patients with UC (Figs. 5.1, 5.2, and 5.3), whereas serosal irregularities can be observed in 80 % of patients with CD, as reported in previous CT and MRI studies [4, 7, 8, 10–13].

Wall stratification is another common finding of UC, observed in approximately 60 % of patients with UC versus 8 % of patients with CD [4, 7, 8, 10–14] (Fig. 5.3). At MRI it may be observed on T2-weighted plain images as a bright wide line within the two dark stripes of the mucosal and muscularis propria, due to increased fat or oedema in the submucosal layer. On T2-weighted images it is possible to further characterize this stratification and to distinguish fat from oedema, by using fat-suppressed imaging, since the fat becomes darker, whereas the oedema remains bright [7–9] (Fig. 5.3d).

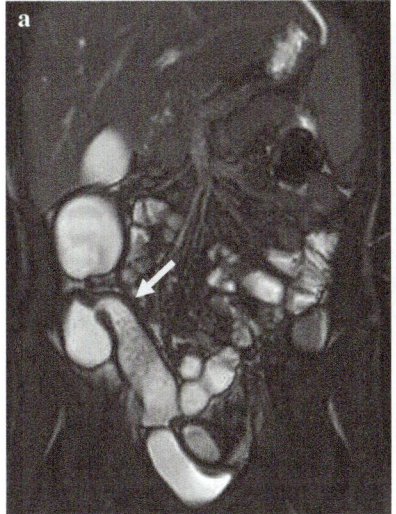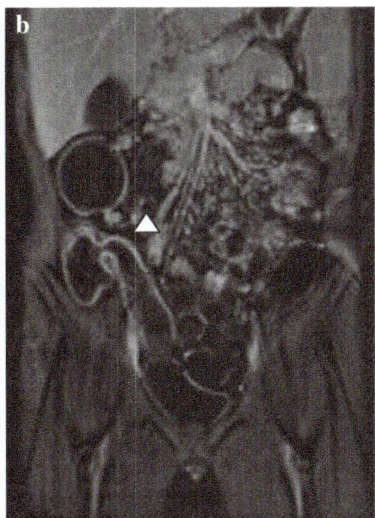

Fig. 5.2 Active ulcerative "pancolitis with back-wash ileitis" in a 10-year-old male with clinical and endoscopic signs of active UC. This patient assumed a biphasic oral contrast agent. **a** The coronal True FISP image shows a mild diffuse thickening of the terminal ileum (*white arrow*), as well as of the *right* colon. **b** T1 VIBE post-contrast fat-saturated coronal MRI image of the same patient shows diffuse wall enhancement of terminal ileum, ileocecal valve and *right* colon, findings consistent with active colitis and backwash ileitis (*white arrow head*)

5.3.2 Morphological Evaluation of UC: Disease Extent and Complications

In UC the intestinal inflammation starts from the rectum and extends proximally, involving progressively different portions of the colon, the descending first, then the transverse and finally the ascending colon and coecum (Fig. 5.1). Occasionally, it may affect the terminal ileum as well, usually in association with a complete colonic involvement, the so-called "back-wash ileitis" (Fig. 5.2). However, while rectosigmoid involvement is present in 95 % of patients at endoscopy, mucosal inflammation of the terminal ileum, the so-called backwash ileitis, is rarely observed [2, 3]. Thanks to its panoramic and multi-planar capability, MRI is usually able to distinguish between a proctitis, a left-sided colitis or a pancolitis, either on axial and coronal planes. Usually, colonic involvement of UC can be better assessed on axial and coronal planes, whereas rectal involvement is better depicted on axial and sagittal planes.

MRI can also detect the loss of haustration in the affected colonic segments (Figs. 5.1f, 5.3g), the presence of strictures and the characteristics of the ileocecal valve and terminal ileum. Loss of colonic haustra is a typical finding of very active phases, while in remission phases haustra can be restored. In advanced chronic fibrotic stages haustra can be permanently lost.

A prominent perirectal fibrofatty proliferation or oedema with widening of the pre-sacral space is another typical morphologic feature of UC (Fig. 5.3b). The complete darkening (suppression) of the perirectal fat signal on T2-weighted fat-suppressed images is a typical feature of longstanding disease. On the other hand, in hyperacute phases of the disease, the perirectal or pericolic fat may show persistent high signal on T2-weighted fat-suppressed images, due to perivisceral oedema (Fig. 5.3c, d). Although perivisceral fibrofatty proliferation is a typical finding of CD rather than of UC, peri-sigmoid or perirectal fat widening is frequently observed in UC as well.

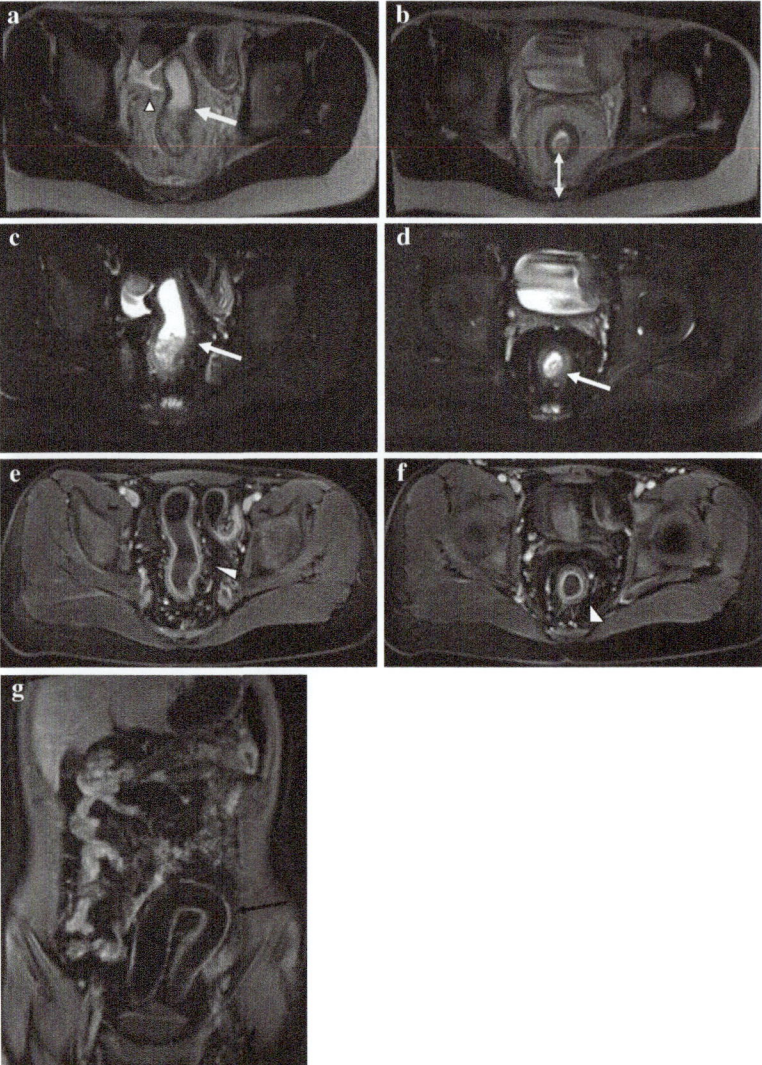

Fig. 5.3 16-year-old patient affected by UC of the left colon, confirmed at endoscopy and histologically proven. **a, b** Axial T2-weighted half-Fourier single-shot turbo spin-echo images acquired at the level of the sigmoid colon and rectum show diffuse thickening and mild stratification of the colonic and rectal wall (*white arrow*), with a minimal amount of perivisceral fluid (*white arrow head*), as well as widening of the pre-sacral fat (*double-headed white arrow*). **c, d** Axial T2-weighted half-Fourier single-shot turbo spin-echo fat-suppressed images show bright signal intensity at the level of the submucosal layer suggesting the presence of submucosal oedema (*white arrow*) rather than fat deposition, thus indicating an active disease. **e, f** T1 VIBE post-contrast fat-saturated axial MRI images demonstrate marked mucosal enhancement (*white arrow head*)↑ confirming the activity of the disease. **g** T1 VIBE post-contrast fat-saturated coronal MRI image demonstrates tubular aspect of the sigmoid colon and post-contrast enhancement due to mucosal inflammation (*black arrow*)

Local enlarged lymph nodes may be detected in the pericolonic fat next to the affected segments in acute phases, although less frequently than in CD. Prominence of vasa recta is another perivisceral finding, frequently observed at the level of inflamed bowel segments. Furthermore, in active UC it is not uncommon to observe minimal amounts of free fluid outside the bowel, suggestive of local serosal inflammation, especially on T2-weighted images (Figs. 5.1d, 5.3a) Active lymph nodes, mesenteric hypervascularity and perivisceral fluid are more frequently observed during the acute phases of the disease [14]. Entero-enteric or entero-adnexal adhesions can also be seen in UC, although less frequently than in CD [7, 8, 10, 14]. Severe fibrotic strictures can be easily detected and graded at MRI on the basis of pre-stenotic lumen distension. They can be considered as benign fibrotic strictures when they are regular and do not show wall thickening or significant wall enhancement. In contrast, neoplastic strictures, a well-known complication of long-standing UC, are characterized by eccentric, marked and irregular wall thickening in the context of an extensively inflamed bowel wall. Nevertheless, MRI cannot be considered a reliable diagnostic tool to distinguish between being and malignant strictures. The detection of neoplastic complications requires endoscopy and biopsy [7, 8].

5.3.3 MRI Differential Diagnosis Between UC and CD

One of the major diagnostic issues in the clinical management of IBD is the differentiation of UC from CD. This is a crucial point in the choice of the appropriate pharmacologic therapy and especially for surgical planning, which is substantially different for the two diseases. Whenever CD presents its typical features, particularly if the small bowel is extensively involved with sparing of the colon, the differentiation from UC is easily achievable. There are, however, several cases where the differential diagnosis may be challenging, particularly in presence of backwash ileitis in UC, or extensive colonic involvement in Crohn's disease.

Involvement of the distal ileum, easily detectable with MRI, is found in over 90 % of adult patients affected by CD and only in a minority of patients affected by backwash in UC [4, 7, 8, 10, 14]. Moreover, backwash ileitis shows milder signs of wall inflammation with respect to CD, and is usually associated with a

continuous involvement of the entire colon, which is quite uncommon in CD (Fig. 5.1). CD of the distal ileum, instead, is usually characterized at MRI by marked wall thickening (>5 mm, <20 mm), marked enhancement, fibrofatty proliferation and enlarged local mesenteric lymph nodes.

On the other hand, involvement of the colon can be found in over 60 % of patients with CD, particularly in paediatric patients [15]. Although it is more frequently associated with involvement of the distal ileum (30−55 % of cases), it may be exclusively limited to the colon in up to 30 % of cases [4, 7, 8, 15]. The rectum may be involved in 50−60 % of patients with CD. Endoscopy and histology alone cannot always differentiate colonic CD from UC, because of the insufficient sampling of the bowel wall layers obtained from biopsy specimens, usually limited to the mucosal and submucosal layers. At MRI, a patchy involvement of the colon or evidence of transmural disease is definitely in favour of the diagnosis of CD rather than of UC. Colonic wall thickening is usually lower in UC than in CD, due to the intramural rather than transmural inflammation; the mean value is 7.8 mm in UC versus 11 mm up to 20 mm in CD [7–13]. Moreover, the outer contour of the colonic wall is regular in patients with UC, whereas mural irregularities are more frequent in CD patients, associated with inflammatory involvement of the mesenteric fat. Fistulas or sinus tracts, adhesions and abscesses are hallmarks of CD and detectable on MRI with high accuracy.

In all these challenging cases, the final diagnosis of IBD should be based on a combination of clinical, MRI, endoscopic and histologic results.

5.4 Assessment of UC Activity: Acute Exacerbations

Endoscopy, together with histology, is currently considered the gold standard for the evaluation of both disease activity and extent in patients with UC [14]. However, evaluation of disease extent by conventional colonoscopy may be contraindicated during severe disease, due to the risk of complications, such as perforation. Moreover, patients frequently refuse repeated colonoscopies due to procedure-related discomfort and due to the inconvenience of extensive bowel cleansing required for an optimal examination.

Therefore, a non-invasive technique such as MRI is desirable in clinical practice, especially during severe exacerbations: (1) to reduce the risk of procedure-related complications and (2) to ensure complete examination of all colonic segments [7, 8, 10, 14].

Assessment of UC activity, like in Crohn's disease, includes evaluation of both mural and extramural signs of inflammation [14–17].

Mural signs of inflammation include bowel wall oedema on T2-weighted images and wall enhancement on T1-weighted ones.

On T2-weighted images, by adding fat suppression, it is possible to distinguish between submucosal fat and oedema, thus characterizing the disease. In acute phases, a persistent bright mucosal and submucosal signal on T2-weighted fat-suppressed images suggests the presence of wall oedema and therefore of active disease [7, 8, 14].

Wall gadolinium enhancement observed on T1-weighted fat-suppressed images is another relevant sign of active UC. The degree of enhancement at the level of the inflamed bowel wall in UC has been related to the degree of inflammatory activity, like in CD [14–18]. According to our experience, in severe active UC a marked wall enhancement is associated with increased wall thickening, whereas less active disease shows moderate wall enhancement and mild thickening [7, 8, 10, 14–18]. In quiescent disease, bowel wall enhancement can be absent. It is important to emphasize that, in our experience, no abnormality can be detected in approximately 10 % of patients with proven quiescent UC [7, 8].

Extramural findings of acute exacerbations are better observed on T2-weighted images, particularly the brightness of the perirectal or pericolic fat due to perivisceral fat oedema and minimal amounts of free fluid outside the bowel, suggesting local serosal inflammation (Figs. 5.1c, 5.3a). Furthermore, both on T1- and T2-weighted fat-suppressed images, local enlarged active lymph nodes and vascular engorgement can be observed.

Recently, several authors [19–22] reported the possibility to assess UC activity with DWI. Oussalah et al. [19] reported 89.4 % sensitivity and 86.6 % specificity in detecting active UC with DW-MRI on a series of 35 patients. They stated that in patients with UC it is possible to replace completely the use of the intravenous contrast medium with MR-DWI in the identification of active inflammatory bowel segments. Another study by Kılıçkesmez et al. [20] reported a good correlation between increased disease activity and decreased ADC values (restricted diffusion) in the rectal wall and in perirectal lymph nodes in 28 patients affected by UC, whereas this correlation was not found at the level of other colonic segments affected by UC. These preliminary results suggest that active wall inflammation in CD determines a restricted diffusion. Further studies are still needed, however, to determine whether and how restricted diffusion correlates with the degree of wall inflammation and why results are not fully concordant in different series [23].

5.5 Role of MRI in the Management of UC: Conclusions

MRI has shown to be extremely valuable in the assessment of disease extent and activity both in adult and paediatric patients affected by UC [15]. To date, it should be considered as a second-level diagnostic tool, with endoscopy still remaining the gold standard.

Indeed, MRI can easily assess the entire colon in presence of fibrotic strictures that may prevent or limit colonoscopy. Furthermore, MRI may be crucial during acute exacerbations of UC, when endoscopy is not recommended due to the high risk of bleeding or perforation. In these cases, the decision of an urgent colectomy may be fully based on the evaluation of the effectiveness of the medical treatment. MRI, being safe and repeatable, can be effectively used to monitor the effects of pharmacologic therapy even in short time intervals, in adult and particularly in paediatric patients [7, 8], thus driving the therapeutic planning in hyperacute severe phases.

Moreover, whenever the endoscopic and pathologic findings are doubtful or controversial, MRI may be helpful in the differentiation between UC and CD, by assessing sparing of the distal ileum and the continuity of colonic involvement.

In conclusion, MRI is becoming the imaging modality of choice in the management of UC, because it enables an accurate diagnosis of the main morphologic features of the disease and assessment of its inflammatory activity, safely and without invasiveness.

References

1. Maccioni F (2012) Feature section: Crohn's disease activity: MRI assessment and clinical implications. Abdom Imaging 37(6):917–920 (Introduction)
2. Jewell DP (1993) Ulcerative colitis. In: Sleisenger MH, Foerdtran JS (eds) Gastrointestinal disease, 4th edn. Saunders, Philadelphia, pp 1305–1330
3. Riddell RH (2000) Patology of idiopatic inflammatory bowel disease. In: Kirsner JB (ed) Inflammatory bowel disease, 5th edn. WB Saunders, Philadelphia, pp 427–447
4. Philpotts LE, Heiken JP, Westcott MA et al (1994) Colitis: use of CT findings in differential diagnosis. Radiology 190:445–449
5. Miner PB (2000) Clinical features, course, laboratory findings, and complications in ulcerative colitis. In: Kirsner JB (ed) Inflammatory bowel disease, 5th ed. W.B. Saunders Co., Philadelphia, pp 299–304
6. Giovagnoni A, Fabbri A, Maccioni F (2002) Oral contrast agent in MRI of the gastrointestinal tract. Abdom Imaging 27:367–375
7. Maccioni F, Colaiacomo MC, Parlanti S (2005) Ulcerative colitis: value of MR imaging. Abdom Imaging 30:584–592
8. Maccioni F (2004) MRI of colitis. In: Chapmann AH (ed) Radiology and imaging of the colon. Springer-Verlag, New York, pp 201–214
9. Maccioni F (2008) Double-contrast magnetic resonance imaging of the small and large bowel: effectiveness in the evaluation of inflammatory bowel disease. Abdom Imaging. doi:10.1007/s00261-008-9482-7
10. Rimola J, Rodríguez S, García-Bosch O et al (2009) Role of 3.0-T MR colonography in the evaluation of inflammatory bowel disease. Radio Graphics 29:701–719
11. Gore RM (1994) Cross sectional imaging of the colon. In: Gore RM, Levine MS, Laufer I (eds) Textbook of gastrointestinal radiology. WB Saunders, Philadelphia, pp 1052–1063
12. Gore RM, Balthazar EJ, Ghahremani GG, Miller FH (1996) CT features of ulcerative colitis and Crohn's disease. AJR 167:3–15
13. Gore RM, Ghahremani GG, Miller FH (1997) Inflammatory bowel disease: radiologic diagnosis. In: Balfe DM, Levie MS (eds) Syllabus of radiological society of north America categorical course in gastrointestinal radiology produced by RSNA publications. RSNA, pp 95–110
14. Ordás I, Rimola J, García-Bosch O (2012) Diagnostic accuracy of magnetic resonance colonography for the evaluation of disease activity and severity in ulcerative colitis: a prospective study. Gut 0:1–7
15. Maccioni F, Viola F, Carrozzo F et al (2012) Differences in the location and activity of intestinal Crohn's disease lesions between adult and paediatric patients detected with MRI. Eur Radiol 22:2465–2477
16. Maccioni F, Viscido A, Broglia L et al (2000) Evaluation of Crohn disease activity with MRI. Abdom Imaging 25:219–228
17. Maccioni F, Bruni A, Viscido A et al (2002) MR imaging in patients with crohn disease: value of T2-versusT1-weighted gadolinium-enhancedMR sequences with use of an OralSuperparamagnetic contrast agent. Radiology 238:517–530
18. Nozue T, Kobayashi A, Takagi Y et al (2000) Assessment of disease activity and extent by magnetic resonance imaging in ulcerative colitis. Pediatr Int 42:285–288
19. Oussalah A, Laurent V, Bruo O et al (2010) Diffusion-weighted magnetic resonance without bowel preparation for detecting colonic inflammation in inflammatory bowel disease. Gut 59:1056–1065
20. Kılıçkesmez O, Soylu A, Yaşar N et al (2010) Is quantitative diffusion-weighted MRI a reliable method in the assessment of the inflammatory activity in ulcerative colitis? Diagn Interv Radiol 6:293–298
21. Oto A, Zhu F, Kulkarni K et al (2009) Evaluation of diffusion-weighted MR imaging for detection of bowel inflammation in patients with Crohn's disease. Acad Radiol 16:597–603

22. Oto A, Kayhan A, Williams JTB et al (2011) Active Crohn's disease in the small bowel: evaluation by diffusion weighted imaging and quantitative dynamic contrast enhanced MR imaging. J Magn Reson Imaging 33:615–624

23. Maccioni F, Patak MA,1 Signore A et al (2012) New frontiers of MRI in Crohn's disease: motilityimaging, diffusion-weighted imaging, perfusionMRI, MR spectroscopy, molecular imaging, and hybrid imaging (PET/MRI). Abdom Imaging 37:974–982

Radiographic and CT Imaging Assessment of Acute Exacerbations and Surgical Complications

6

Sonia Ippolito, Massimo Tonolini and Chiara Villa

6.1 Acute Severe Colitis and Toxic Megacolon

Although ulcerative colitis (UC) is a chronic inflammatory disease of the large bowel, approximately 15 % of patients experience at least a severe attack during their lifelong course [1, 2].

According to the most recent European Crohn's and Colitis Organization (ECCO) guidelines, classification of UC based on severity is useful for clinical practise and dictates patient management. Currently, the definition "acute severe colitis" (ASC) should be preferred to the vague term "fulminant" colitis. Systemic symptoms such as anorexia, malaise, vomiting and fever are characteristic of acute attacks, along with severe intestinal symptoms such as increased stool frequency, bloody diarrhoea and/or urgency. Conversely, massive rectal haemorrhage is an exceptional occurrence [1, 2].

Disease activity in UC is most usually staged according to the Consensus criteria by Truelove and Witts, which take into account the number of bloody stools per day, heart rate, temperature, haemoglobin and C-reactive protein. Criteria for ASC include six or more bloody bowel movements per day, plus fever >37.8 °C, pulse >90/sec or haemoglobin <10.5 g/dL. Alternatively, clinicians may choose to adopt the Modified Montreal Criteria, or the Mayo score which include stool frequency along with rectal bleeding, mucosal features and physician's global assessment of performance status [1, 2].

A potentially life-threatening condition, ASC represents an indication for hospital admission for intensive treatment including intravenous steroids, and may lead to the need for urgent colectomy if clinical improvement does not occur within a week [3, 4].

The very recent 2013 joint ECCO and ESGAR (European Society of Gastrointestinal and Abdominal Radiology) consensus guidelines recognized a decreasing status of abdominal radiographs in favour of ultrasound and multi-detector CT (MDCT) in the triage of patients with idiopathic inflammatory bowel diseases (IBD) and acute abdomen. However, although often unremarkable due to the limited assessment of the mucosal outline, supine and upright plain films still have value and should be recommended as potentially useful in the initial assessment of patients with suspected ASC, followed by flexible sigmoidoscopy which allows to confirm active disease. Phosphate enema preparation before sigmoidoscopy is safe, but probably best avoided if the colon is dilated.

S. Ippolito (✉) · M. Tonolini · C. Villa
Radiology Department, "Luigi Sacco" University Hospital, Via G.B. Grassi 74, 20157 Milan, Italy
e-mail: ippolito.sonia@hsacco.it

M. Tonolini
e-mail: mtonolini@sirm.org

C. Villa
e-mail: chiara.villa@hotmail.it

M. Tonolini (ed.), *Imaging of Ulcerative Colitis*,
DOI: 10.1007/978-88-470-5409-7_6, © Springer-Verlag Italia 2014

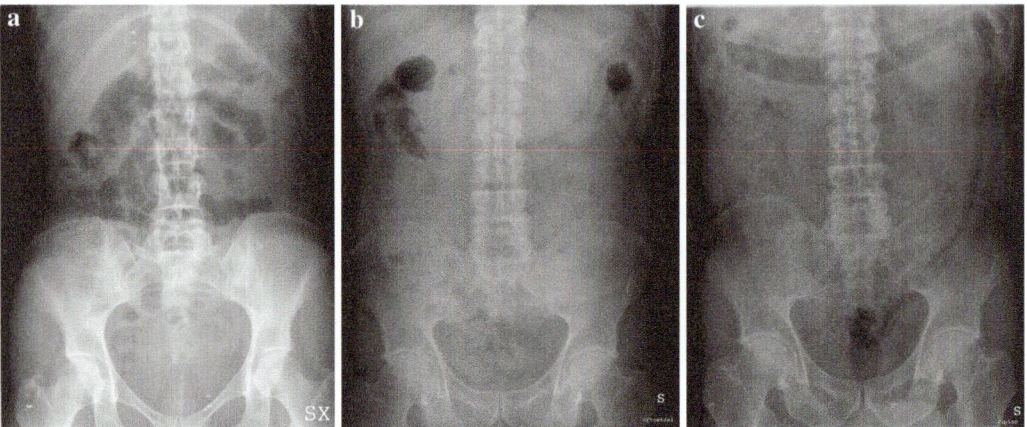

Fig. 6.1 In a 40-year-old woman with clinically severe UC confirmed by sigmoidoscopy, disease distribution up to the hepatic flexure is grossly estimated on supine plain abdominal radiograph (**a**), with moderately dilated transverse colon. In a 56-year-old man with ASC, upright (**b**) and supine (**c**) plain films show extensive involvement of the transverse, descending and rectosigmoid colon by mural thickening with abnormal mucosal pattern, absent haustra and some foreshortening

Conversely, full colonoscopy during acute ASC is not advised [1, 2, 5].

The two key radiological issues to be considered when interpreting abdominal films in patients with known UC and suspected ASC include assessment of intestinal dilatation, and of the gross disease distribution. Concerning the former issue, since intraluminal gas tends to accumulate with increasing disease severity, a diffuse or segmental colonic dilatation >5.5 cm in transverse diameter correlates strongly with mucosal ulceration at endoscopy, and is associated with a 75 % need for colectomy. Furthermore, ileus (represented by three or more small bowel loops distended with gas) is associated with a 50 % colectomy rate [1–4].

The next issue to be considered relates to the fact that the longitudinal extent of UC disease influences both prognosis and patient management, particularly regarding the choice of oral and/or topical therapy. Disease distribution of UC is classified according to the Montreal criteria, taking into account the maximal macroscopic extent of disease at colonoscopy or double-contrast barium enema, in three stages defined as proctitis (with involvement limited to the rectum), left-sided (distal to the splenic flexure) and extensive colitis (proximal to the splenic flexure, including pancolitis). Radiographically, the proximal distribution of disease broadly correlates with the most distal presence of faecal residues (Fig. 6.1). Sometimes, mural thickening may be appreciated radiographically, either with the "thumbprinting sign" corresponding to thickened oedematous haustra appearing as endoluminal finger-like marginal indentations at contours of the colonic wall, or as diffuse haustral loss and "mucosal islands" of irregular internal pattern (Fig. 6.1). Furthermore, radiographic follow-up may be useful, since persistent distension in ASC correlates with poor response to therapy, and may support the decision to perform urgent surgery [1–4].

The classical definition of toxic megacolon (TM) indeed represents the end of the spectrum of ASC, and is defined as a total or segmental non-obstructive dilatation of the colon (>6 cm), associated with systemic toxicity that occurs in approximately 5 % of patients with ASC. In recent decades, earlier diagnoses, improved intensive medical treatment and timely surgery, have dramatically reduced the incidence of TM complicating UC. At imaging, TM may be suggested by extensive, unchanging colonic distension with loss of haustral pattern resulting from transmural ulceration with destruction of the myenteric plexus and apparent mural thickening with frequently appreciable "thumbprinting sign". The entire colon may be involved, but changes are usually most apparent in the transverse colon which is the least-dependent segment of the colon. Early colectomy is indicated when no improvement is observed within 24 h [3–5].

In a recent study, CT findings did not differ significantly between patients who required surgery and those who were not operated, and had therefore a minor impact on the decision to perform colectomy in patients with ASC [6]. Conversely, our personal experience confirms that MDCT is increasingly requested to further investigate patients with acute presentations of known IBD. Although with the drawback of ionizing radiation and intravenous contrast

medium, MDCT quickly provides a comprehensive assessment of the entire abdominal and pelvic organs, peritoneum, intra-abdominal fat and lymph nodes. Furthermore, routine image reconstruction (Fig. 6.2) along coronal and sagittal planes provides a panoramic visualization of intestinal abnormalities, associated mesenteric and extraintestinal changes or complications, with sub-millimetre spatial resolution reproducing the classical orientation of double-contrast barium enema which is familiar to most surgeons.

Despite being primarily a mucosal disease, UC is commonly characterized at MDCT by mural colon thickening, which is of moderate entity (6–9 mm), circumferential and symmetric in the majority of cases (Figs. 6.2, 6.3 and 6.4). Wall thickening is positively associated with

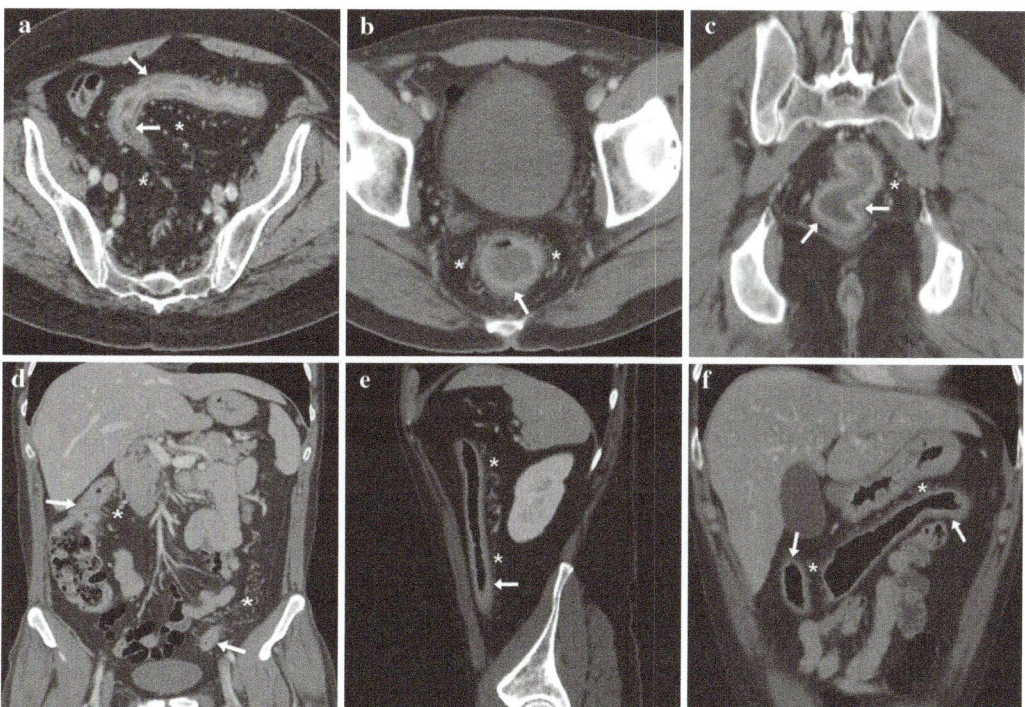

Fig. 6.2 A 75-year-old male with known UC and acute abdominal pain. Urgent contrast-enhanced MDCT (**a**) is requested to exclude other co-existent intra-abdominal diseases, and allows to effectively stage proctosigmoiditis by showing moderate mural thickening with stratified "water halo" appearance (*arrows*), associated proliferation and hypervascularization of pericolonic

fat (*). In a different patient, a 49-year-old male, similar MDCT changes (**b–f**) are detected throughout the rectum, sigmoid, descending and transverse colon, up to the transition between hepatic flexure and ascending tract, leading to diagnose pancolitis. In both patients, perforation, peritoneal effusion and abscesses are confidently excluded, thus allowing medical treatment

endoscopic, clinical and histopathological severity [5, 7, 8].

Colonic mural stratification is seen in approximately 70 % of cases. During ASC, the stratified appearance is due to mucosal hyperenhancement (corresponding to endoscopic erosion and ulceration changes) coupled with thickened oedematous submucosa. The resulting "target" or "water halo" sign best seen in transverse planes, characterized by a low-attenuation intermediate ring, represents acute inflammatory disease (Figs. 6.2 and 6.3). Most usually, UC changes show a continuous distribution from the rectum (which is spared in 4 % of cases only) to the left-sided (Fig. 6.2) or the entire colon (Fig. 6.3) [7–10].

Conversely, the "fat halo sign" mural stratification with a fat-density intermediate ring corresponding to widening and adipose infiltration of the colon submucosa that separates the bowel mucosa from the outer soft-tissue muscularis propria and serosa, represents chronic stages of UC [9–11].

Additionally, extraintestinal MDCT changes characteristically observed in UC include proliferation of pericolonic fat with hyperaemia and vascular engorgement, a slightly increased attenuation (10–20 HU) compared to normal abdominal fat due to oedema and inflammation, often containing nodular densities corresponding to enlarged lymph nodes (Figs. 6.2, 6.3, 6.4 and 6.5), most consistently identifiable in the perirectal area [7, 12].

As such, urgent-setting contrast-enhanced MDCT improves assessment of both colonic dilatation (Fig. 6.4) and longitudinal distribution of UC disease, as compared to plain radiographs. Due to the high correlation of mural stratification and mucosal hyperenhancement with clinical and endoscopic severity, contrast-enhanced MDCT may be helpful in ASC as an alternative to endoscopy, to confirm disease severity [7].

Furthermore, at our Department urgent-setting water enema MDCT (WE-MDCT) with limited or no bowel preparation has been attempted and generally proven useful in

Fig. 6.3 A 65-year-old woman with clinical diagnosis of acute severe UC (ASC). Contrast-enhanced MDCT effectively depicts severe enhancing mural thickening of the rectosigmoid colon (*arrowheads* in **a**) and associated perivisceral fat changes (*), plus stratified oedematous mural thickening throughout the descending, transverse and *right* colon (*arrows* in **b**, **c**, **d**), allowing diagnosis of severe pancolitis and obviation of endoscopy

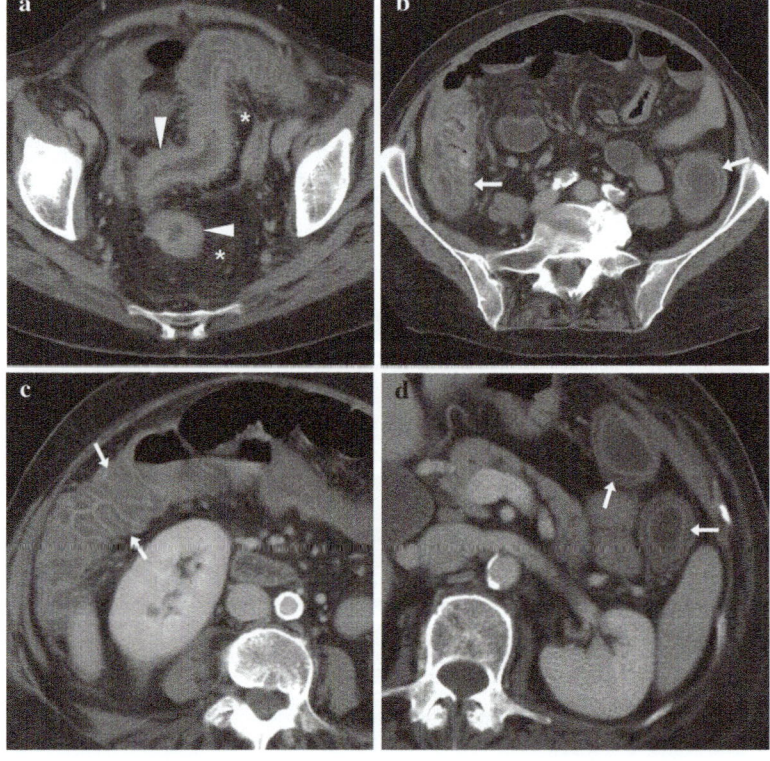

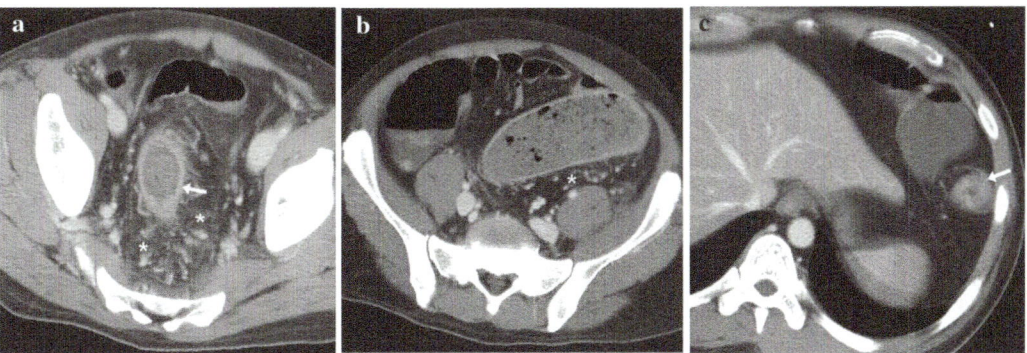

Fig. 6.4 A 42-year-old male with clinical suspicion of ASC. Contrast-enhanced MDCT visualizes moderate colonic mural thickening (*arrows*) of the rectosigmoid (**a**)and descending colon, up to the splenic flexure (detail in **c**), with segmental dilatation of the sigmoid colon (in **b**) and associated perivisceral fat changes (*). Failure to respond to medical treatment led to perform urgent colectomy

Fig. 6.5 A 69-year-old female with known UC, investigated with WE-MDCT using limited bowel preparation during an acute disease exacerbation. The rectum and sigmoid colon show circumferential mural thickening (*arrowheads*) with "water halo sign" appearance (**a**) and associated perirectal fat proliferation (*). The upstream colon appears well-distended with normal mural thickness and some endoluminal faecal residues (**c, d**). Findings are consistent with *left-sided* ASC and allow obviating the need for endoscopy (Reprinted from *Open Access* Ref. no. [13])

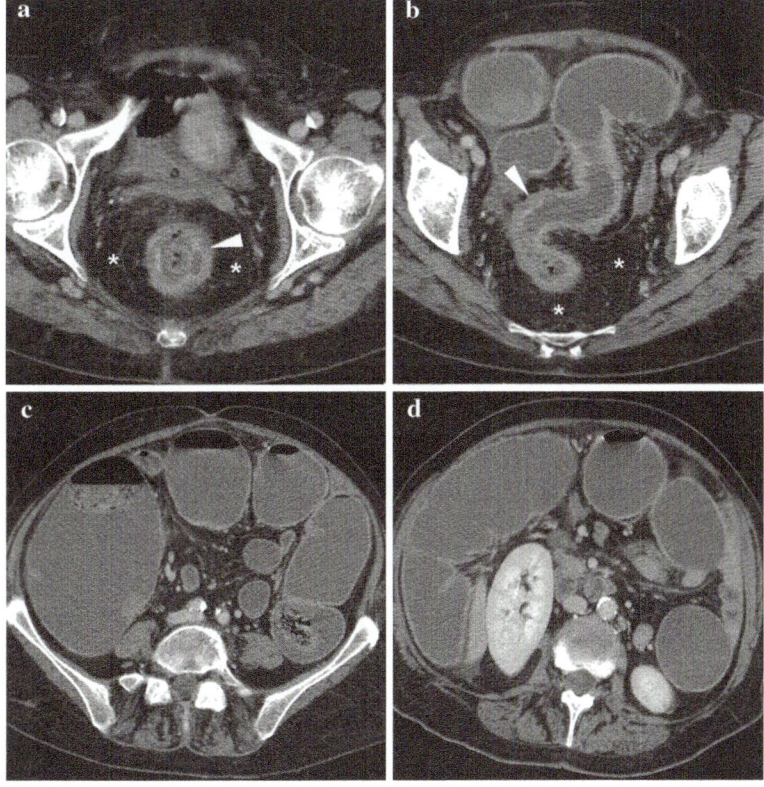

selected patients with ASC. Performed with the same technique as described in Chap. 4 of this volume, WE-MDCT is not recommended when TM, free perforation and acute peritonitis are clinically suspected and/or radiographically detected [13].

Despite the presence of faecal residues, which is the rule when bowel preparation is limited or avoided, in our experience WE-MDCT further improves assessment of the bowel wall in its full-thickness and therefore confirmation of disease activity. Furthermore, WE-MDCT

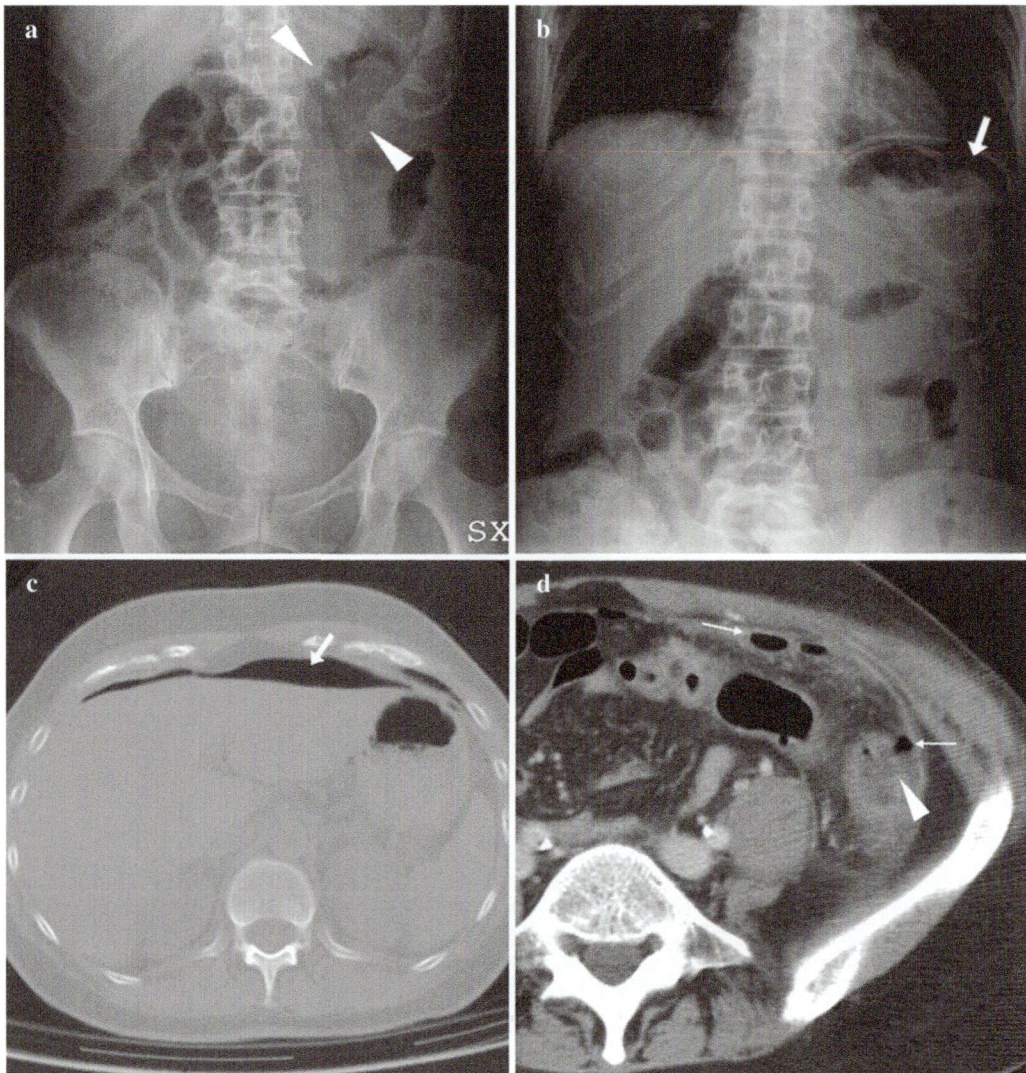

Fig. 6.6 A 45-year-old woman with unremarkable past medical history, presents to emergency department because of severe abdominal pain. Found peritonitic at physical examination, she then reveals relapsing bowel symptoms since some months earlier, which were not further investigated. Supine (**a**) and upright (**b**) plain abdominal radiographs show *left*-sided subphrenic air (*arrow*) consistent with perforation, and mural thickening with "thumbprinting sign" (*arrowheads*) perceptible along the transverse colon. Contrast-enhanced MDCT confirms free intraperitoneal air (*arrow* in **c**, viewed at lung window), and directly identifies perforation site as a focal discontinuity (*arrowhead* in **d**) in the moderately thickened wall of the descending colon, from which gas bubbles (*thin arrows*) originate. Surgical exploration and further workup confirmed colonic perforation, caused by previously undiagnosed UC

allows an easy identification of the transition between the involved large bowel that is not completely distended despite pharmacological hypotonisation, and the upstream healthy segments that usually appear well-distended with non-thickened walls and preserved haustral folds (Fig. 6.5) that is crucial for a correct longitudinal distribution staging of UC, with the aim to allow a correct therapeutic choice. Therefore, the use of WE-MDCT can obviate endoscopy which is contraindicated or risky because of increased risk of perforation [13].

Finally, as extensively discussed in Chap. 9 of this book, when interpreting MDCT studies obtained in patients with ASC the veins (particularly the spleno-portal-mesenteric system) should be scrutinized for opacification defects consistent with thrombosis. Venous thrombi are often multiple, peripheral and occlusive, whereas central thrombi in the main veins tend to be non-occlusive [14–17].

6.2   Perforation

Colonic perforation is the second most serious complication of ASC, usually associated with toxic dilatation, inappropriately delayed surgery, colonoscopy or missed UC diagnosis (Fig. 6.6), and is associated with a 50 % mortality [3, 4].

Although free intraperitoneal air may be detected on upright abdominal radiographs, emergency MDCT is warranted due to its high accuracy in predicting site of gastrointestinal perforation, by considering the supra- or infra-mesocolic distribution of intra-abdominal air and wall thickening in the involved bowel segment. At MDCT, even minimal extraluminal gas bubbles are confidently detected. Direct identification of the bowel wall discontinuity indicating perforation site is often possible by careful review of MDCT images (Fig. 6.6) [18, 19].

6.3   Superimposed Infection

Whereas TM and perforation are very rarely encountered nowadays, the incidence of infective complications is reportedly increasing. In patients with an established diagnosis of UC, microbial testing for superimposed *Clostridium difficile* and Cytomegalovirus (CMV) is recommended in cases of ASC or refractory relapse. Although uncommon, pseudomembranous colitis (PMC) is increasingly encountered because of the widespread use of broad-spectrum

antibiotics, which leads to unopposed overgrowth of enterotoxin-releasing *C.difficile*. PMC represents a growing concern in hospitalized patients, particularly those with decreased immune function and history of prolonged antibiotic therapy, because it is associated with increased morbidity and mortality. Furthermore, CMV reactivation in immunosuppressed patients with UC may contribute to refractory or worsen ASC [1–4].

Imaging findings of infectious colitis invariably include bowel wall thickening of variable degree with usual "water halo" appearance, and thus significantly overlap with those observed in ASC. At MDCT, superimposed infection may be suggested by extensive colonic involvement from the caecum to the rectum by severe colonic wall thickening (at least 1–1.5 cm), often associated with fascial, presacral fluid and ascites (in up to 40 % of cases) which are rather unusual findings in patients with UC [9, 10].

References

1. Dignass A, Eliakim R, Magro F et al (2012) Second European evidence-based consensus on the diagnosis and management of ulcerative colitis part 1: definitions and diagnosis. J Crohns Colitis 6:965–990
2. Stange EF, Travis SP, Vermeire S et al (2008) European evidence-based consensus on the diagnosis and management of ulcerative colitis: definitions and diagnosis. J Crohns Colitis 2:1–23
3. Dignass A, Lindsay JO, Sturm A et al (2012) Second European evidence-based consensus on the diagnosis and management of ulcerative colitis part 2: current management. J Crohns Colitis 6:991–1030
4. Travis SP, Stange EF, Lemann M et al (2008) European evidence-based Consensus on the management of ulcerative colitis: current management. J Crohns Colitis 2:24–62
5. Panes J, Bouhnik Y, Reinisch W et al (2013) Imaging techniques for assessment of inflammatory bowel disease: joint ECCO and ESGAR evidence-based consensus guidelines. J Crohns Colitis 7:556-85
6. da Luz Moreira A, Vogel JD, Baker M et al (2009) Does CT influence the decision to perform colectomy in patients with severe ulcerative colitis? J Gastrointest Surg 13:504–507
7. Patel B, Mottola J, Sahni VA et al (2012) MDCT assessment of ulcerative colitis: radiologic analysis with clinical, endoscopic, and pathologic correlation. Abdom Imaging 37:61–69

8. Gore RM, Balthazar EJ, Ghahremani GG et al (1996) CT features of ulcerative colitis and Crohn's disease. AJR Am J Roentgenol 167:3–15

9. Horton KM, Corl FM, Fishman EK (2000) CT evaluation of the colon: inflammatory disease. Radiographics 20:399–418

10. Thoeni RF, Cello JP (2006) CT imaging of colitis. Radiology 240:623–638

11. Ahualli J (2007) The fat halo sign. Radiology 242:945–946

12. Regge D, Neri E, Turini F et al (2009) Role of CT colonography in inflammatory bowel disease. Eur J Radiol 69:404–408

13. Norsa AH, Tonolini M, Ippolito S et al (2013) Water enema multidetector CT technique and imaging of diverticulitis and chronic inflammatory bowel diseases. Insights Imaging 4:309-320

14. Nahon S, Cadranel JF, Chazouilleres O et al (2009) Liver and inflammatory bowel disease. Gastroenterol Clin Biol 33:370–381

15. Shen B, Remzi FH, Lavery IC et al (2008) A proposed classification of ileal pouch disorders and associated complications after restorative proctocolectomy. Clin Gastroenterol Hepatol 6:145–158 (quiz 124)

16. Remzi FH, Fazio VW, Oncel M et al (2002) Portal vein thrombi after restorative proctocolectomy. Surgery 132:655–661 (discussion 661–662)

17. Ball CG, MacLean AR, Buie WD et al (2007) Portal vein thrombi after ileal pouch-anal anastomosis: its incidence and association with pouchitis. Surg Today 37:552–557

18. Ghekiere O, Lesnik A, Millet I et al (2007) Direct visualization of perforation sites in patients with a non-traumatic free pneumoperitoneum: added diagnostic value of thin transverse slices and coronal and sagittal reformations for multi-detector CT. Eur Radiol 17:2302–2309

19. Hainaux B, Agneessens E, Bertinotti R et al (2006) Accuracy of MDCT in predicting site of gastrointestinal tract perforation. AJR Am J Roentgenol 187:1179–1183

Cross-Sectional Imaging Mimics of Ulcerative Colitis

Massimo Tonolini

Nowadays, CT performed on multidetector scanners (MDCT) is extensively used to investigate patients with acute abdominal complaints. In most cases, MDCT provides prompt and reliable detection of acute abnormalities involving the peritoneum, parenchymal organs, biliary and urinary tracts, retroperitoneum and vascular structures, allowing timely triage between medical and surgical treatment [1].

Additionally, MDCT is almost universally accepted as the preferred modality to investigate suspected acute conditions involving the intestines, that can assess severity and longitudinal extent of enterocolitis, differentiate from malignancy and exclude complications requiring surgery such as perforation, abscess formation or gangrene. The key advantages of MDCT include universal availability, acquisition speed, routine multiplanar image reformation and comprehensive demonstration of colonic wall, perivisceral fat and adjacent structures [1, 2].

In the general population, MDCT identification of colonic mural thickening greater than 5 mm is highly predictive of colonic pathology (72.3 % sensitivity, 64–96.5 % specificity) and therefore warrants further investigation with colonoscopy. In published series, CT detection of colonic thickening in non-selected patients allowed to diagnose previously unknown neoplasms, infections, ischaemia, diverticulitis or chronic inflammatory bowel diseases (IBD), although with a non-negligible portion of normal cases [3–5].

Because of the large number of urgent-setting MDCT studies daily performed, the detection of cross-sectional imaging appearances suggesting colitis is a not-uncommon occurrence in most busy radiology departments. Although the true thickness of the colonic wall is best assessed with hypotonization and retrograde water enema, as described in Chap. 4 dealing with CT examination technique, a pathologic mural thickening can be suggested in most cases when urgent MDCT is acquired without peroral and rectal intraluminal contrast. In a distended colon, the mural thickness should not exceed 3–4 mm, whereas in a collapsed segment the normal wall thickness can reach 4–5 mm [2, 6].

In patients without an established diagnosis of chronic IBD, CT imaging features suggesting Ulcerative colitis (UC) may be observed in a varied spectrum of acute or chronic colonic disorders.

7.1 Crohn's Disease

The diagnosis of Crohn's disease (CD) is usually made on the basis of clinical features, endoscopy with biopsy samples. Despite the considerable overlap existing between colonic Crohn's disease (CD) and UC features, the identification of

M. Tonolini (✉)
Radiology Department, "Luigi Sacco" University Hospital, Via G.B. Grassi 74, 20157 Milan, Italy
e-mail: mtonolini@sirm.org

M. Tonolini (ed.), *Imaging of Ulcerative Colitis*,
DOI: 10.1007/978-88-470-5409-7_7, © Springer-Verlag Italia 2014

mural abnormalities in both small and large bowel shifts the diagnosis towards the former entity (Fig. 7.1). When only the colon is affected, the degree and geographic distribution of bowel wall thickening should be considered to suggest the most probable underlying IBD condition. UC is typically distal, left-sided or diffuse, whereas isolated right colon involvement is exceptional. CD most usually involves the distal ileum and proximal colon, with a narrow ileocecal valve. Conversely, "backwash ileitis" associated with UC may appear as dilatation of the terminal ileal loop with a gaping valve and shaggy thin walls. Although a diffuse colitis pattern may be observed, left-sided colon CD is rare. Rectal involvement is characteristic of UC and very uncommon in CD patients [2, 6, 7].

Both chronic IBD conditions involve a significant degree of colon mural thickening, which is usually more pronounced in CD (mean 11 mm) than in UC (7−8 mm). Furthermore, wall thickening in UC is symmetric and continuous, whereas in granulomatous CD colitis it usually appears eccentric or asymmetric, with

segmental distribution and spared "skip" tracts (Fig. 7.1) [2, 6, 7].

The thickened colon wall in IBD usually demonstrates a stratified pattern. The "target" or "water halo" sign refers to a triple-layered appearance of the bowel when seen in a plane perpendicular to its main axis, with an outer soft-tissue ring representing the muscularis mucosa and serosa, a middle ring of intermediate density caused by the thickened oedematous submucosa and an inner ring of enhancing, inflamed mucosa (Fig. 7.2). Although unspecific, this CT sign is invariably associated with acute bowel injury (usually from an infectious or inflammatory cause), and virtually excludes malignancy [2].

The water halo sign should be differentiated from the "fat halo" sign , which is seen more often (61 %) in patients with UC, than in CD colitis (8 %). The thickened bowel wall demonstrates three layers with different CT density: the inner soft-tissue attenuation layer represents the enhancing mucosa, the intermediate fat-density (-65 Hounsfield Units (HU) to -10 HU) layer

Fig. 7.1 48-year-old male with multifocal ileo-colic Crohn's disease. Water enema multidetector CT including multiplanar image reformations shows short non-distensible bowel segments with stratified mural thickening involving the splenic flexure (*arrows* in **a** and **b**), descending colon (*arrowheads* in **b** and **c**) and distal ileum (*thin arrows* in **c** and **d**)

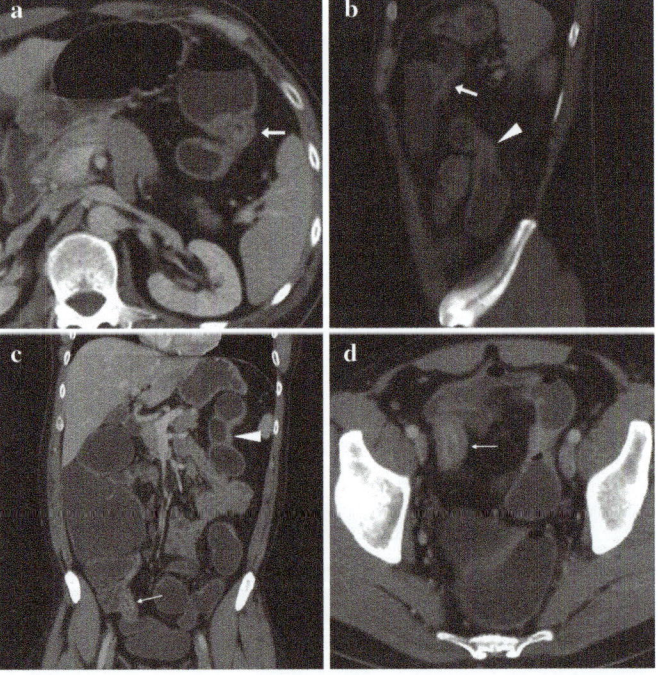

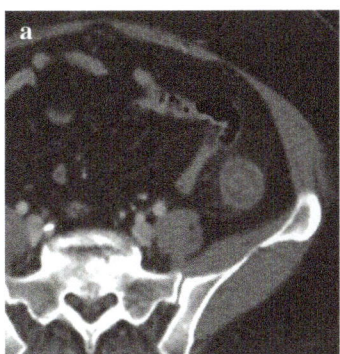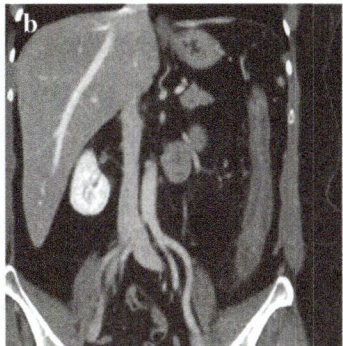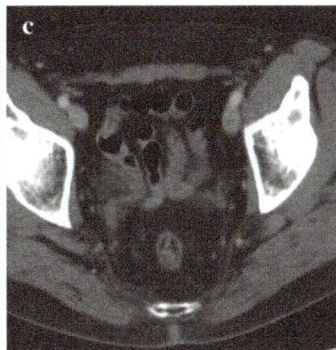

Fig. 7.2 Urgent contrast-enhanced MDCT (**a**, **b**) in a 65-year-old woman with clinical suspicion of acute diverticulitis shows extensive involvement of the descending colon by circumferential mural thickening with "target sign" stratification due to oedematous submucosa, consistent with acute infectious colitis. In another 50-year-old male patient with known chronic ulcerative colitis, the rectum (**c**) shows mural stratification with "fat halo" sign corresponding to submucosal adipose deposition, associated with mesorectal fat proliferation

results from widening and fatty infiltration of the submucosa, and the outer soft-tissue layer corresponds to the muscularis propria and serosa (Fig. 7.2). This CT sign may be observed on both unenhanced and post-contrast acquisitions because of the marked differences in tissue attenuation, and should suggest a diagnosis of IBD with fatty infiltration of the submucosa, particularly UC. Alternatively, this sign has been reported in patients undergoing cytoreductive chemotherapy and in graft-versus-host disease [6–8].

Other helpful features to distinguish UC from CD colitis involve the pericolonic structures. In UC, proliferation of perirectal fat is frequently observed, with a slightly increased attenuation (10−20 HU) compared to the normal mesenteric fat, and traversed by nodular and streaky soft-tissue attenuation structures (Fig. 7.2). In CD, fibrofatty proliferation and lymphadenopathy involves the mesentery, often in an extensive way. Observed more frequently in association with CD, is the "comb sign" corresponding to tubular opacities aligned on the mesenteric side of the involved bowel segment corresponding to hypervascularity with vascular dilatation, tortuosity and wide spacing of the vasa recta, secondary to increased flow related to the acute inflammation. Finally, internal fistulas and abscess collections are relatively specific to CD [6, 7, 9].

7.2 Colonic Infections

Cross-sectional imaging appearances similar to those described in IBD may be observed in many different colonic infections, that are usually diagnosed clinically, on the basis of stool cultures and endoscopy. Significant overlap exists between the imaging appearances of most colonic infections, since they all share the common MDCT features of mural thickening, most usually with a stratified appearance due to submucosal oedema and enhanced inflamed mucosa, associated with pericolonic fat stranding and variable ascites (Figs. 7.3, 7.4) [2, 6].

Sometimes, the involved causative organism may be suggested by the distribution of CT abnormalities along the colon. A diffuse ("pancolitis") involvement is observed with pseudomembranous colitis (PMC), cytomegalovirus and *Escherichia coli* infections. Resulting from *Clostridium difficile* overgrowth following antibiotic therapies, PMC produces the most severe degree of colon wall thickening, with prominent target/water halo appearance, associated with mild ascites and pericolonic fat infiltration (Fig. 7.4). Although insensitive, the suggestive "accordion" sign refers to positive intraluminal contrast entrapped between the thickened haustral folds [2, 6].

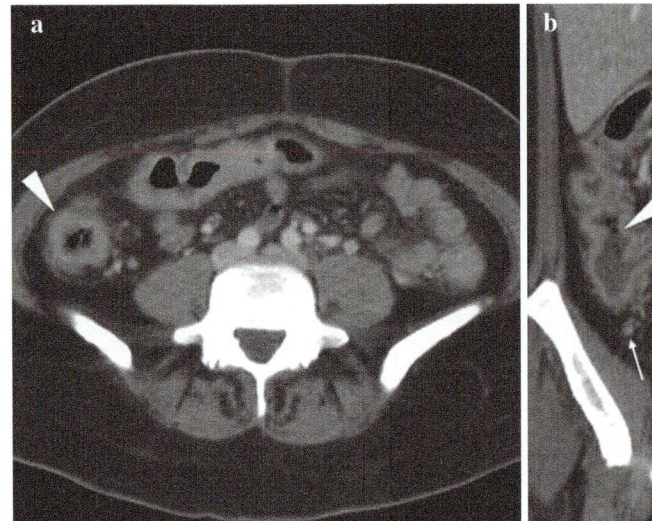
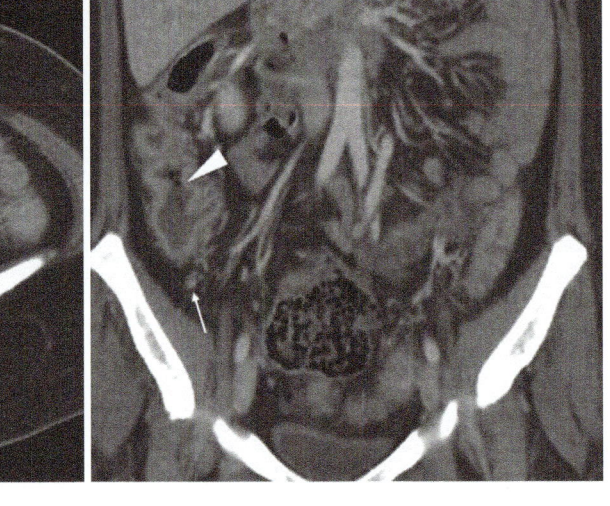

Fig. 7.3 42-year-old woman from East Europe suffering from acute febrile infectious enteritis with bloody stools. Axial (**a**) and coronal reformatted (**b**) contrast-enhanced MDCT images show mural thickening of the *right* colon with hyperenhancing mucosa (*arrowheads*), mild pericolonic inflammatory fat stranding with tiny lymph nodes

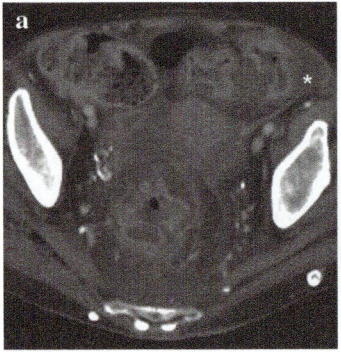
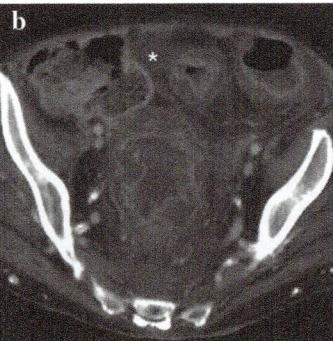
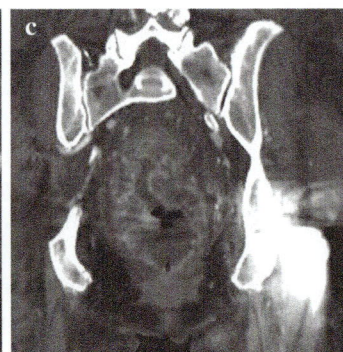

Fig. 7.4 Elderly 81-year-old woman with *Clostridium difficile* pseudomembranous colitis following antibiotic therapy. Axial (**a**, **b**) and coronal (**c**) contrast-enhanced MDCT images show severe rectosigmoid colon thickening with prominent "target sign" due to severely oedematous submucosa and strong mucosal enhancement, associated with perivisceral fat stranding and moderate ascites (*)

An ileal and right colon predominance suggests *Salmonella*, *Yersinia*, tuberculosis or amoebiasis, with the latter two conditions increasingly encountered in patients from endemic countries. Conversely, a left-sided predominance may be related to *Shigella* infection. Sexually transmitted infections such as gonorrhoea, herpesvirus and *Chlamydia* tend to involve typically the rectosigmoid. Although the distribution and mural changes in severe colonic infections such as PMC may mimic those of UC or colonic CD, the key

associated findings of peritoneal effusion and pericolonic changes suggest an acute intestinal inflammation and are rather unusual in patients with chronic IBD (Fig. 7.4) [2, 6].

7.3   Ischaemic Colitis

Ischaemic colitis (IC) is increasingly encountered in the ageing Western population, and may result from a sudden loss of arterial or venous

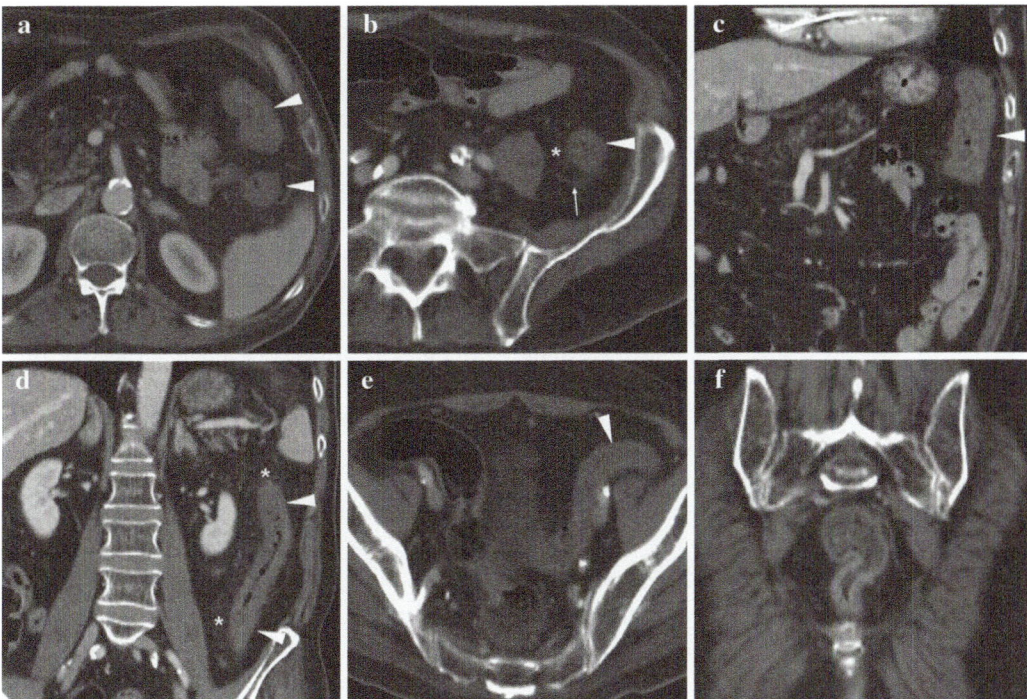

Fig. 7.5 70-year-old man with cardiac pacemaker, abdominal pain and profuse bloody diarrhoea. Multiplanar contrast-enhanced MDCT images (a–d) reveal nondistended *left* flexure, descending and sigmoid colon with circumferential mural thickening and poor enhancement (*arrowheads*), associated with perivisceral fat inflammation (*) and minimal ipsilateral fascial fluid (*thin arrow*). Rectal sparing was noted (**e**, **f**). Surgical exploration confirmed extensive colonic ischaemia, treated with left colectomy

blood flow or conversely from a low-flow state such as in cardiac arrhythmias. Whereas intestinal infarction due to total vascular occlusion is a dramatic event causing severe acute abdomen and shock, non-transmural IC with reperfusion presents with minor abdominal pain and rectal bleeding and with CT features that may be easily misinterpreted as chronic IBD. IC may be diffuse or segmental, more commonly involving the left-sided colon when due to hypoperfusion (Fig. 7.5). Additionally, watershed areas of the colon such as the splenic flexure and rectosigmoid are particularly susceptible to ischaemia, because they are situated at the borders of major vascular territories. MDCT imaging shows circumferential, symmetric wall thickening with haustral fold enlargement, the target sign due to oedema or otherwise high attenuation indicating intramural haemorrhage, pericolonic stranding, fascial and/or peritoneal fluid (Fig. 7.5). Coupled with appropriate clinical history, the absent involvement of the rectum favours ischaemia over UC [2, 6].

7.4   Diverticulitis

Diverticulitis occurs in up to 25–33 % of patients with colonic diverticular disease, which is a highly prevalent condition in the general population in Western countries, and represents a common cause of acute abdominal complaints that increases in frequency with advancing age. Acute diverticulitis most usually involves the sigmoid and distal descending colon, and in 20 % of cases may be further complicated by perforation with abscess formation, or fistulization to adjacent organs, particularly the urinary bladder, sometimes the vagina, uterus and small bowel [10, 11].

Currently, MDCT represents the mainstay modality to investigate suspected diverticulitis, yielding a very high accuracy for identification of acute pericolonic fat inflammation, contained or free perforation and allowing confident identification of features (such as perivisceral abscesses and extraintestinal gas collections) that indicate high risk of failure and recurrence with conservative treatment [10, 11]. The usual CT findings observed in diverticulitis include colonic hypersegmentation and wall thickening due to muscular hypertrophy and spasm, associated with diverticular outpouchings of the colonic wall, usually filled by air or enterolith, increased density and hypervascularization of the inflamed perivisceral fat and fascial thickening close to the pelvic side. The key to distinguish diverticulitis from other inflammatory conditions such as IBD and IC is the presence of diverticula in the involved segment (Fig. 7.6) [2, 6, 10–12].

7.5   Miscellaneous Conditions

Chronic radiation injury of the large bowel results from radiation-induced endoarteritis, and most commonly affects the sigmoid colon following treatment of pelvic uro-gynaecological malignancies. Although this entity shows non-specific appearances including wall thickening, the fat halo sign, pelvic fat proliferation and increased density, the diagnosis is usually made on the basis of positive treatment history [6].

Another uncommon condition that appears as an acute colitis on cross-sectional imaging is non-steroidal anti-inflammatory drug (NSAID) drug-related injury, which is underestimated and very scarcely reported in the medical literature despite the extensive use of medications in the general population and its potential seriousness [13–18].

Mostly affecting elderly people and patients on long-term therapy, NSAID colitis may result from administration of oral, rectal and topical

Fig. 7.6 80-year-old overweight woman with acute diverticulitis and bloody diarrhoea. Urgent contrast-enhanced MDCT shows extensive mural thickening of the recto-sigmoid (**a**–**c**) and descending colon (**d**) with uniformly thickened walls due to oedematous submucosa. Multiple small-sized diverticula are appreciated in the sigmoid tract (*arrowheads*). Imaging exclusion of perforation and abscess collections allowed conservative treatment

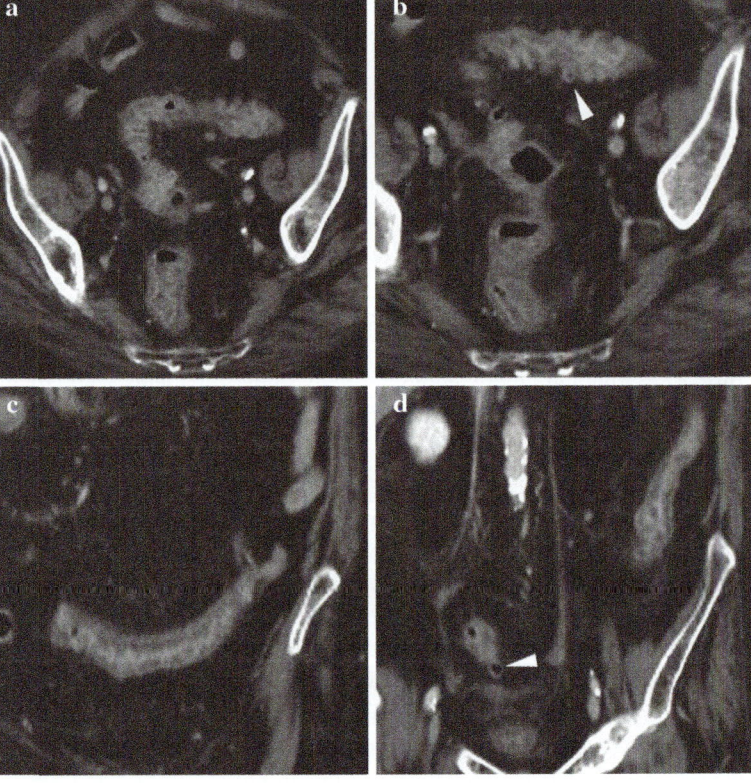

preparations prescribed to treat a wide range of symptoms [16, 19]. Although its pathogenesis and natural history are poorly understood, NSAID-induced colitis present with diffuse abdominal pain, diarrhoea, lower gastrointestinal bleeding or alternatively in a subacute form with weight loss, malaise and iron-deficiency anaemia [13–17, 19].

This condition may be diagnosed on the basis of positive drug history, consistent endoscopic, imaging and pathological changes and associated negative stool cultures and insignificant biochemical abnormalities. Unfortunately, endoscopy and histology from biopsy specimens are unspecific in most cases; as a result misinterpretation as CD, UC or IC is not exceptional [14, 17, 19].

In NSAID-induced colitis, cross-sectional imaging findings include circumferential mural thickening with a "water halo" appearance due to low-attenuation oedematous submucosa, predominantly involving the right colon and distal ileum, decreasing abnormalities along the transverse, descending and sigmoid tracts and rectal sparing [13, 15, 18].

Finally, non-inflammatory intestinal abnormalities are commonly encountered (31−35 % prevalence) in patients with chronic liver disease Benign intestinal wall oedema and thickening in cirrhosis occurs secondary to hypoalbuminemia, portal hypertension or a combination of both, and significantly correlates with the severity of liver impairment measured by Child-Pugh grades, with portal hypertension signs such as splenomegaly and varices score, and with serum albumin levels [20, 21]. Large bowel mural thickening is predominantly limited to the right colon (in up to two-thirds of cases), may sometimes involve the transverse (19 %) and descending (12 %) portions or be multi-segmental in 17 % of patients (Fig. 7.7) [20–22].

Imaging studies with endoscopic correlation revealed that more than half of cirrhotic patients with CT colonic abnormalities have a normal

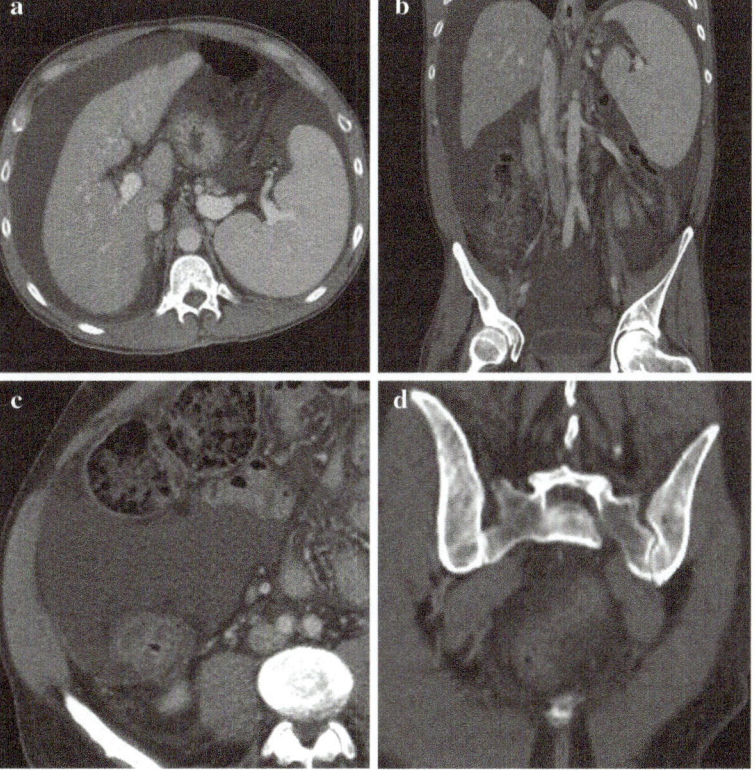

Fig. 7.7 53-year-old male with decompensated liver cirrhosis investigated with MDCT after, with limited ultrasound assessment. Contrast-enhanced images show hepatosplenomegaly and ascites (**a**), *right* colon involvement by severe mural thickening with enhancing mucosa and oedematous submucosa, closely resembling an acute infectious-inflammatory colitis (**b,c**). Similar changes of a lesser entity are observed in the rectosigmoid colon (**d**)

intestinal mucosa at colonoscopy. Non-specific changes such as diffuse mucosal oedema, increased vascularity and chronic teleangiectasia are commonly encountered (44 %) in cirrhotic patients, but these benign changes do not require any further investigation or intervention [21].

Since patients with chronic liver disease are frequently investigated with CT, these incidental colonic findings may give rise to diagnostic dilemmas [20, 21]. CT identification of concentric thickening, particularly involving the right colon with well-demarcated wall layers, associated with history of chronic liver disease, portal hypertension and hypoalbuminemia, does not warrant further investigation or follow-up and colonoscopy may be avoided in this population [21, 22].

References

1. Leschka S, Alkadhi H, Wildermuth S et al (2005) Multi-detector computed tomography of acute abdomen. Eur Radiol 15:2435–2447
2. Thoeni RF, Cello JP (2006) CT imaging of colitis. Radiology 240:623–638
3. Wolff JH, Rubin A, Potter JD et al (2008) Clinical significance of colonoscopic findings associated with colonic thickening on computed tomography: is colonoscopy warranted when thickening is detected? J Clin Gastroenterol 42:472–475
4. Nicholson BD, Hyland R, Rembacken BJ et al (2011) Colonoscopy for colonic wall thickening at computed tomography: a worthwhile pursuit? Surg Endosc 25:2586–2591
5. Eskaros S, Ghevariya V, Diamond I et al (2009) Correlation of incidental colorectal wall thickening at CT compared to colonoscopy. Emerg Radiol 16:473–476
6. Horton KM, Corl FM, Fishman EK (2000) CT evaluation of the colon: inflammatory disease. Radiographics 20:399–418
7. Gore RM, Balthazar EJ, Ghahremani GG et al (1996) CT features of ulcerative colitis and Crohn's disease. AJR Am J Roentgenol 167:3–15
8. Ahualli J (2007) The fat halo sign. Radiology 242:945–946
9. Madureira AJ (2004) The comb sign. Radiology 230:783–784
10. Werner A, Diehl SJ, Farag-Soliman M et al (2003) Multi-slice spiral CT in routine diagnosis of suspected acute left-sided colonic diverticulitis: a prospective study of 120 patients. Eur Radiol 13:2596–2603
11. Poletti PA, Platon A, Rutschmann O et al (2004) Acute left colonic diverticulitis: can CT findings be used to predict recurrence? AJR Am J Roentgenol 182:1159–1165
12. Ambrosetti P, Becker C, Terrier F (2002) Colonic diverticulitis: impact of imaging on surgical management—a prospective study of 542 patients. Eur Radiol 12:1145–1149
13. Aftab AR, Donnellan F, Zeb F et al (2010) NSAID-induced colopathy. A case series. J Gastrointestin Liver Dis 19:89–91
14. Puspok A, Kiener HP, Oberhuber G (2000) Clinical, endoscopic, and histologic spectrum of nonsteroidal anti-inflammatory drug-induced lesions in the colon. Dis Colon Rectum 43:685–691
15. Katsinelos P, Christodoulou K, Pilpilidis I et al (2002) Colopathy associated with the systemic use of nonsteroidal antiinflammatory medications. An underestimated entity. Hepatogastroenterology 49:345–348
16. Gleeson MH, Davis AJ (2003) Non-steroidal anti-inflammatory drugs, aspirin and newly diagnosed colitis: a case-control study. Aliment Pharmacol Ther 17:817–825
17. Evans JM, McMahon AD, Murray FE et al (1997) Non-steroidal anti-inflammatory drugs are associated with emergency admission to hospital for colitis due to inflammatory bowel disease. Gut 40:619–622
18. Ballinger A (2008) Adverse effects of nonsteroidal anti-inflammatory drugs on the colon. Curr Gastroenterol Rep 10:485–489
19. Geramizadeh B, Taghavi A, Banan B (2009) Clinical, endoscopic and pathologic spectrum of non-steroidal anti-inflammatory drug-induced colitis. Indian J Gastroenterol 28:150–153
20. Ormsby EL, Duffield C, Ostovar-Sirjani F et al (2007) Colonoscopy findings in end-stage liver disease patients with incidental CT colonic wall thickening. AJR Am J Roentgenol 189:1112–1117
21. Guingrich JA, Kuhlman JE (1999) Colonic wall thickening in patients with cirrhosis: CT findings and clinical implications. AJR Am J Roentgenol 172:919–924
22. Baba Y, Hokotate H, Inoue H et al (2001) Correlations between colonic wall thickening in patients with virally induced cirrhosis on CT and clinical status. J Comput Assist Tomogr 25:786–791

Hepato-Bilio-Pancreatic Complications of Ulcerative Colitis

8

Giovanni Pompili, Alice Munari, Alessandro Campari and Gianpaolo Cornalba

8.1 Introduction

Extraintestinal manifestations (EIMs) occur in up to 30 % of patients affected by ulcerative colitis (UC) or Crohn's disease. Hepato-bilio-pancreatic (HBP) complications are one of the most common EIMs in patients with UC, together with musculoskeletal and mucocutaneous manifestations. Different from other EIMs, diseases involving the HPB system typically do not correspond to UC activity and may adopt an independent course irrespective of the intestinal inflammation [1]. This association has different pathogenic mechanisms: in some patients liver disease is related to the IBD itself, in others it is caused by their pharmacological treatment, while in some other patients, neither of these elements appears to be involved [2]. As suggested by Navaneethan et al. [1], four different kinds of mechanisms can be identified:

(1) *diseases possibly associated with a shared pathogenetic mechanism with IBD,* including primary sclerosing cholangitis (PSC), small-duct PSC/pericholangitis, PSC/autoimmune hepatitis overlap, IgG4-associated cholangitis, cholangiocarcinoma (CCA), acute and chronic "idiopathic" pancreatitis related to IBD;

(2) *diseases with parallel structural and physiological changes seen with IBD,* including cholelithiasis, portal vein thrombosis and hepatic abscess;

(3) *diseases related to adverse effects associated with treatment of IBD,* including drug-induced hepatitis, pancreatitis (purine-based agents) or liver cirrhosis (methotrexate), reactivation of hepatitis B, and biologic agent-associated hepatosplenic T cell lymphoma;

(4) less common HPB manifestations described in patients with IBD, *possibly associated with them,* including autoimmune pancreatitis (AIP), primary biliary cirrhosis, fatty liver, granulomatous hepatitis and amyloidosis.

PSC is by far the most important condition associated to UC. Other HBP manifestations including pericholangitis, steatosis, chronic hepatitis, cirrhosis and gallstone formation are more common in UC than in the general population. In most cases, presentation involves abnormal liver function tests with a predominantly obstructive pattern, rather than symptoms or signs of HBP disease. Whereas ultrasound may be used as a screening modality, Magnetic resonance cholangiopancreatography (MRCP) is

G. Pompili (✉) · A. Munari · A. Campari · G. Cornalba
Diagnostic and Interventional Radiology, S. Paolo Hospital, A. Di Rudinì, Milan, Italy
e-mail: gpompili@fastwebnet.it

A. Munari
e-mail: aliceam555@gmail.com

A. Campari
e-mail: alessandro.campari@unimi.it

G. Cornalba
e-mail: gianpaolo.cornalba@unimi.it

M. Tonolini (ed.), *Imaging of Ulcerative Colitis,*
DOI: 10.1007/978-88-470-5409-7_8, © Springer-Verlag Italia 2014

now established as the diagnostic test of choice for PSC. When MRCP is normal, it is probably safer and more diagnostic to perform liver biopsy rather than diagnostic Endoscopic retrograde cholangiopancreatography (ERCP). The use of ERCP may serve to treat dominant strictures by dilatation and/or stenting. Serology is needed to identify specific autoimmune or infectious causes. Drug hepatotoxicity should be always considered and excluded [3].

8.2 Bile Ducts Involvement

8.2.1 Primary Sclerosing Cholangitis

Primary sclerosing cholangitis is a chronic, progressive, cholestatic hepatobiliary disorder of unknown aetiology characterized by inflammation, fibrosis and strictures in medium- and large-sized ducts of the biliary tree [3, 4].

8.2.1.1 Epidemiology and Prevalence of IBD-RCU During PSC

PSC affects young and middle-aged patients, between the third and fifth decades of life with a 2:1 male predominance, particularly those with an underlying IBD [1]. PSC is rare in the general population. Data from Olmsted County (USA) in the year 2000 identified 20.9 cases of PSC per 100,000 of the population in men and 6.3 per 100,000 in women [5]. The association of PSC and IBD was first described in 1965 [6] and it is commonly stated that PSC represents the most common HPB manifestation of IBD. Approximately 70–80 % of patients with PSC have concomitant IBD and 1.4–7.5 % of patients with IBD will develop PSC during the course of their disease [1]. UC is the main IBD involved: the prevalence of PSC was reported to be 2–7.5 % of patients with UC and, in patients with PSC and IBD, 85–90 % have UC, with the latter having either Crohn's colitis or Crohn's ileocolitis [1].

8.2.1.2 Impact of Co-existing PSC/IBD on Behaviour and Course of the Disease

UC associated with PSC has been found to have characteristic features and it should be considered as a separate clinical entity, using the term PSC-IBD [7]. Patients with PSC-UC, compared with UC patients without a concomitant PSC, usually demonstrate a higher prevalence of rectal sparing, backwash ileitis, pancolitis, colorectal neoplasia and overall a poorer survival [8, 9]. It is relevant that the presence of PSC was shown to be an independent risk factor for the development of colorectal dysplasia/cancer in patients with UC (odds ratio 6.9) [10, 11]. This risk affects the ECCO guidelines and the surveillance schedules, which recommend annual colonoscopy from PSC diagnosis, instead of the standard 2-year interval. Vice versa, there is no conclusive evidence that the natural history and the clinical features of PSC differ between patients with and without associated IBD. It has been noted that in patients with PSC-IBD liver disease shows abnormal liver function tests (LFTs), while PSC patients without IBD were more likely to present with jaundice, itch and fatigue. Moreover, patients with PSC-IBD frequently have combined intra- and extra-hepatic bile duct strictures than those without IBD (82 vs. 46 %) [12]. There is no correlation between the severity of UC and the severity of PSC. The risk for development of colorectal cancer (CRC) persists even after patients have orthotopic liver transplantation (OLT); similarly colectomy does not appear to modify the course of PSC. However, OLT for PSC or PSC-associated cholangiocarcinoma (CCA), may affect the clinical course of UC, as corticosteroids and other immunosuppressive agents used following OLT might improve a co-existing UC.

8.2.1.3 Pathogenesis

The aetiology and pathogenesis of PSC are still unknown. The association of PSC with IBD and other autoimmune diseases with multiple humoral and cellular immune abnormalities suggested the influence of immunopathogenic mechanism and genetic susceptibility on the aetiology of PSC [13, 14]. A variety of autoantibodies were detected in patients with PSC, including antinuclear antibodies (ANA), smooth muscle antibodies (SMA) and anti-perinuclear cytoplasmic antibody (pANCA). However, the role of these autoantibodies for the diagnosis and differential diagnosis of PSC or PSC-IBD has not been established. Multiple genetic factors associated with susceptibility have been reported and immunogenetic studies have identified a number of key HLA haplotypes associated with PSC. HLA-B8/DR3 haplotype is particularly common in patients with PSC and UC and infrequent in patients with PSC alone.

8.2.1.4 Prognosis

Despite treatment PSC is generally progressive and its prognosis is poor. Median survival without OLT after diagnosis is approximately 12 years [4]. PSC extension into the hepatic parenchyma with bridging fibrosis and ultimately cirrhosis represents advanced disease. OLT is the treatment of choice for patients with end-stage liver disease due to PSC, which may recur after transplantation in up to 20 % of patients [15]. The major cause of mortality is the occurrence of CCA, which is significantly increased in patients with PSC, with a 10–15 % lifetime risk. This risk is higher in patients with associated IBD than those with PSC alone [4]. Unfortunately, CCA often presents in advanced stage and has poor prognosis, with only 5–11 months of average survival [16]. CCA usually arises around the common hepatic duct and its bifurcation and less commonly in the common duct, gallbladder, cystic duct and intrahepatic ducts with equal frequency [17]. CCA should be suspected in patients with rapid biochemical deterioration and progressive jaundice, weight loss and abdominal pain [14, 16].

8.2.1.5 Diagnosis

Up to 45 % of patients with PSC are asymptomatic at diagnosis and develop symptoms over time [14]. Fatigue, pruritus, jaundice, abdominal

pain and weight loss can be seen in 10–15 % of patients at presentation. These symptoms develop in 60 % of patients over the course of the disease. Diagnosis is based on the association of four diagnostic criteria:

(1) a cholestatic pattern on LFTs, mainly represented in elevation of alkaline phosphatase and serum bilirubin;
(2) radiological findings of intra- and/or extrahepatic anomalies of the bile ducts using ultrasound, CT, MRCP and ERCP;
(3) histological signs of biliary disease;
(4) clinical history of histologically demonstrated IBD.

If no other aetiology can be identified for liver abnormality, the diagnosis of PSC is done in the presence of two of these four criteria including at least one histological or radiological positive finding. There is a weak correlation among biological, histological and radiographic findings: histological diagnosis is often inconclusive and the most common histological features, fibrous obliterating cholangitis and paucity of bile ducts, are absent in more than two-thirds of the bioptic specimens due to the heterogeneous distribution of lesions within the liver. Histological specimen usually shows an aspecific fibrosing inflammation and is only used to confirm a suspicion of PSC [2].

8.2.1.6 Diagnosis with Imaging: Which Is the Best Method ?

The simplest, less expensive and most widely available option to study the liver is abdominal US. It is very effective for revealing a dilated biliary tree and very accurate for measuring the duct diameter. Moreover, US is useful in visualizing mass lesions of the liver. However, abdominal US lacks specificity for the dilatation of the biliary tree, and is not able to evaluate strictures [18]. A standard multidetector computed tomography (MDCT) scan can demonstrate with good sensitivity dilated biliary segments, but again, it is relatively non-specific and cannot reveal whether it was caused by structuring cancer or a benign condition such as PSC. Moreover, although strictures of large bile ducts result in easily visible dilation, strictures affecting small biliary ducts are often not visible [18]. On the other hand, CT scan can detect hepatic and pancreatic lesions, particularly mass lesions, with high sensitivity and provide structural evaluation of the liver and the entire abdomen for other abnormalities. Endoscopic retrograde cholangiopancreatography has been considered for years as the gold standard for diagnosis of PSC [19, 20]. By the way the evaluation of the diameter alteration of bile ducts in PSC can result in false-positive diagnoses when incomplete biliary tract distension mimics ductal irregularities and in false-negative diagnosis when high-grade strictures cause inadequate opacification of intrahepatic ducts [21]. ERCP is an invasive procedure associated with risk of severe complications, such as sepsis, pancreatitis, bowel perforation and cholangitis [22]. Diagnostic ERCP is associated with a major complication rate of 1.3 % and a mortality rate of 0.21 % [23]. Risk of cholangitis is increased in PSC patients because a biliary tree with multiple strictures promotes stasis and perforation due to ductal sacculations and rigidity. On the other hand, ERCP offers the opportunity to obtain tissue samples, particularly by biliary brushings. Moreover, ERCP advantages include the chance to perform treatment by means of endoscopic balloon dilatation and stenting, which may lead to an improvement of biliary drainage, symptoms and biochemical profiles. Percutaneous transhepatic cholangiography (PTC) is not usually used as a diagnostic tool, due to its invasive nature, but it is very useful in the interventional radiology field, to solve high biliary strictures (far from the Vaterian papilla) which are unreachable with ERCP. The percutaneous approach produces clinical and biochemical improvements equal to those brought about by endoscopic management. It is indicated when endoscopy had failed or is technically impossible, as in case of surgically altered anatomy [24]. Magnetic resonance cholangiopancreatography (MRCP) represents an application of MR technology that permits an evaluation of the biliary tract without the use of contrast material or invasive instrumentation and thereby avoids the complications of ERCP and PTC [20, 25]. A recent meta-analysis [23] confirms an excellent accuracy of MRCP for the diagnosis of PSC (ROC curve of 0.91) with a high sensitivity (0.86) and very high specificity (0.94). The results of meta-analysis on cost-minimization and cost-effectiveness studies show that the initial diagnostic test in a patient suspected of having PSC should be MRCP, while ERCP/PTC should only be performed when therapeutic ballooning/stenting is needed [26]. MRCP technique varies on the basis of the imaging unit available, but every MRCP study should include at least:

(a) breath-hold heavily T2w images: thick sections with single-shot fast spin echo technique; thin sections acquired on oblique coronal plane to long axis of the extrahepatic bile duct;

(b) T2w SE sequence on transverse and/or coronal plane including structures from the porta hepatis to the Vaterian papilla;

(c) T1w GE fat-suppressed sequence on transverse plane including structures from the porta hepatis to the whole pancreas.

MRCP images are rapidly acquired and the entire bile tract is visualized in less than 20 s. Different from ERCP, MRCP depicts bile ducts in their natural degree of distension, using as contrast medium the bile itself, hyperintense in heavily T2-weighted images. As a consequence, strictures, biliary sludge and stones, which normally may limit opacification with contrast medium, do not limit the evaluation of bile ducts. Multiplanar MR displays images virtually in any plane and their feature is comparable to that of ERCP or PTC (Fig. 8.1) [25]. Other advantages of MRCP, compared with ERCP, consist in being a less expensive technique, avoiding ionizing radiation and anaesthesia, being less operator-dependent and, when combined with axial section T1w and T2w, allowing evaluation of extra biliary duct pathology. Limitations to MRCP are the presence of stent or air-filled bile ducts from previous ERCP and concentrated bile due to stasis causing signal loss and reduced ducts visualization [27]. False-positive diagnosis with MRCP occurs in cirrhosis that results in a distortion of the intra-hepatic bile ducts, mimicking intrahepatic ductal changes similar to those of PSC. False-negative diagnosis with MRCP occurs when PSC is almost limited to third and fourth order bile ducts [21].

8.2.1.7 Diagnosis with Imaging: Cholangiographic Signs

Imaging demonstration of diffuse, multifocal strictures and irregularities involving the medium-sized intrahepatic and/or medium- or large-sized extrahepatic ducts is the gold standard for diagnosing PSC (Fig. 8.1). Cholangiographic abnormalities include multiple strictures, saccular dilatations and irregularity of ductal margins [28]. Randomly distributed, short (1–2 mm), annular intrahepatic strictures alternating with normal or slightly dilated segments produce a beaded appearance. Some authors suggest "beading appearance" (Fig. 8.2) as the presence of more than three strictures with alternating dilatation along a bile duct [29]. Strictures usually occur at the bifurcation of ducts and are out of proportion to upstream ductal dilatation [14]. As the fibrosing process worsens, strictures increase and the ducts

become obliterated: at this stage the peripheral ducts cannot be visualized at ERCP ("pruned tree" appearance) but are well detected by MRCP as well as complications such as diverticular like extroflessions, saccular dilatations, webs (focal 1–2 mm thick areas of incomplete circumferential narrowing) and biliary stones (Fig. 8.3) [14, 27]. Both intra- and extra-hepatic ducts are usually involved. Lesions are limited to intrahepatic ducts in less than 20 % of cases, and to extra-hepatic ducts in less than 10 %. Cystic duct, gallbladder and pancreatic duct involvement have been described [2]. MRCP and ERCP show different results depending on the involved biliary tract. ERCP ensures a better detection of choledocic irregularities and diameter alterations. The injection of contrast medium through the catheter placed in prepapillary position causes distension of the choledocic tract, allowing better opacification [30]. However, retrograde opacification shows the proximal end of a stricture but may fail to demonstrate the ductal anatomy distal to the stricture. MRCP shows better in visualizing periferical intra-hepatic ducts distal to severe strictures (Fig. 8.4) [30]. Intra-hepatic ductal dilatation is defined by the presence of intra-hepatic bile ducts with diameter

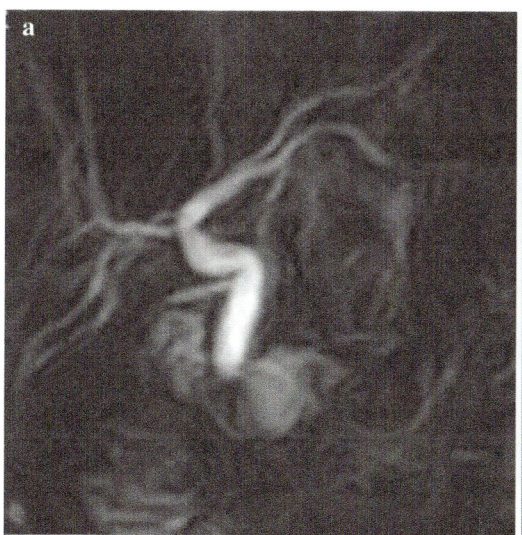
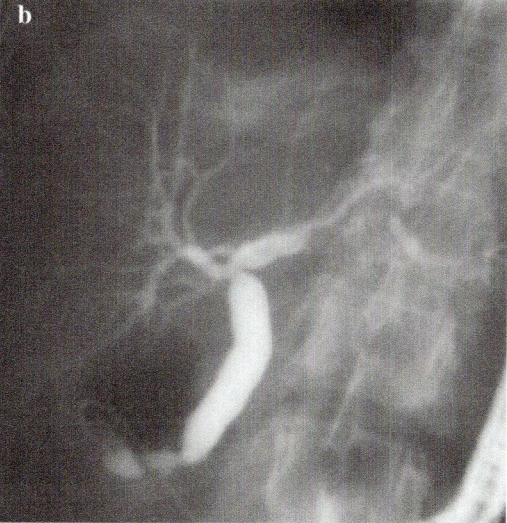
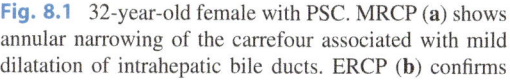

Fig. 8.1 32-year-old female with PSC. MRCP (**a**) shows annular narrowing of the carrefour associated with mild dilatation of intrahepatic bile ducts. ERCP (**b**) confirms MRI statements. Distal choledocic annular stenosis, missed at MRCP, is also depicted

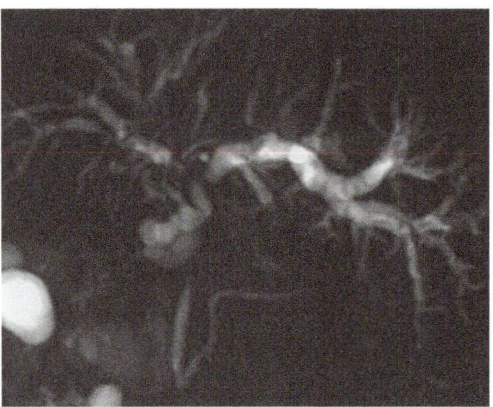

Fig. 8.2 46-year-old female. MRCP shows typical features of PSC with multiple strictures involving intra-hepatic bile ducts, giving a beaded-like appearance and a main stricture on the common bile duct

equal or superior to that of central ducts or major than 3 mm. A mild dilatation has a maximum diameter of 4 mm, a moderate dilatation has a diameter between 4 and 6 mm and a severe dilatation is larger than 6 mm. There is evidence that the level of intra-hepatic bile duct visualization with MRCP is different between patients affected or not by PSC. In healthy individuals,

central ducts contain enough bile in order to be detected by MRCP, while it is difficult to image minor ducts because they contain a negligible amount of bile. In PSC patients peripheral ducts can be imaged more effectively with MRCP in terms of dilatation, which is secondary to strictures in central ducts. Consequently, a good visualization of peripheral intrahepatic bile ducts with MRCP can alarm the radiologist about the presence of a stricture [27]. It should be noted that areas of minimal narrowing may be missed at MRCP and length of stenosis may be overestimated [30].

8.2.1.8 Differential Diagnosis

Before the diagnosis of PSC is established, processes that mimic PSC at cholangiography must be excluded. Cholangiographic findings are similar in primary and secondary cholangitis [28] and a differential diagnosis on the basis of common imaging is not possible. It is not usually possible to differentiate PSC from chronic bacterial cholangitis, parasitic infection of the bile, cholangitis related to acquired immunodeficiency syndrome (AIDS), IgG4-associated cholangitis, infiltrative diseases (such as

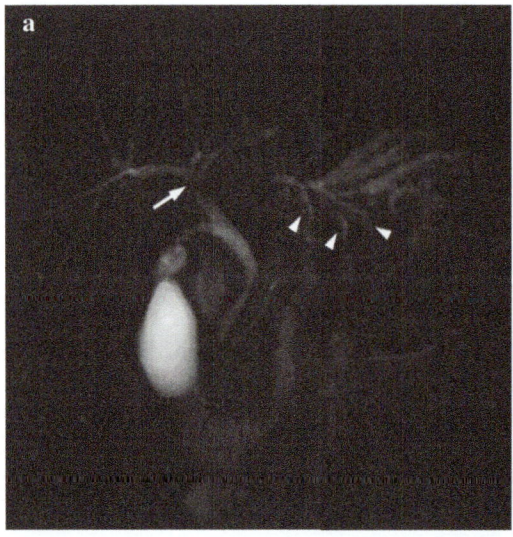
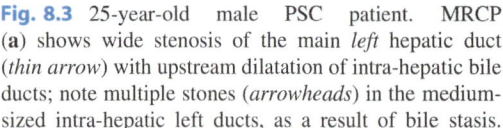
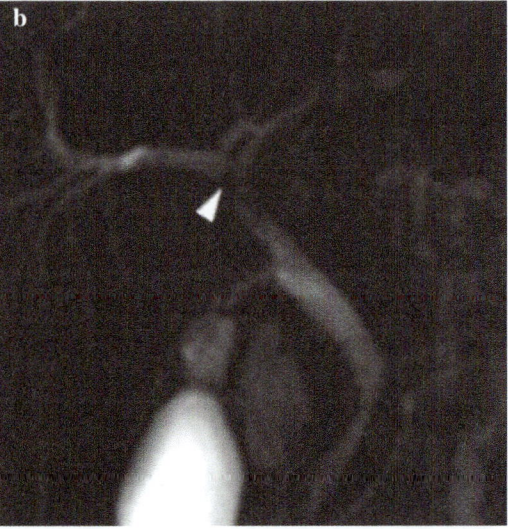

Fig. 8.3 25-year-old male PSC patient. MRCP (**a**) shows wide stenosis of the main *left* hepatic duct (*thin arrow*) with upstream dilatation of intra-hepatic bile ducts; note multiple stones (*arrowheads*) in the medium-sized intra-hepatic left ducts, as a result of bile stasis. Detailed view (**b**) shows focal (1.8 mm) incomplete circumferential stenosis, consistent with "web" of the proximal aspect of the *right* main duct (*arrowhead*). Irregular narrowing of the margins of the common bile duct is also depicted

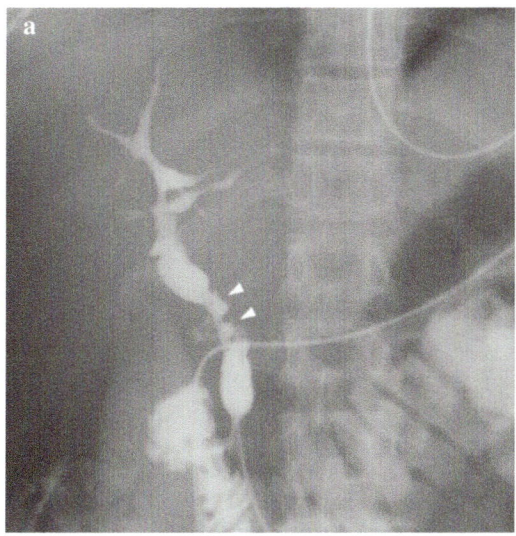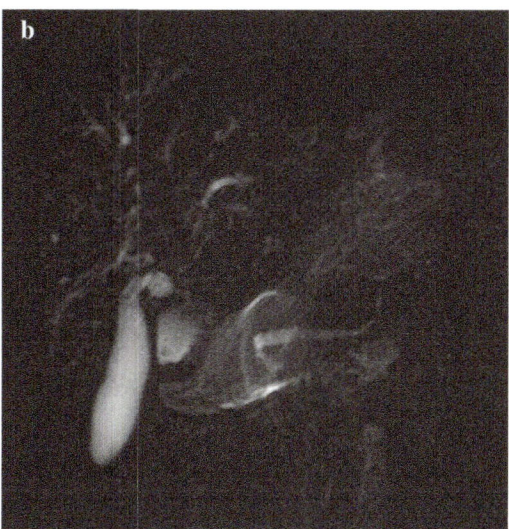

Fig. 8.4 28-year-old male PSC patient. Cholangiography (**a**) shows multiple irregular high-grade stenosis and saccular dilatations of the common bile duct (*arrowheads*). Peripheral ducts could not be visualized at the periphery of the liver ("pruned tree" appearance) because of upstream ducts stenosis. On the other hand, MRCP (**b**) enables to appreciate medium-sized intra-hepatic ducts, affected by diffuse, multifocal strictures. The common bile duct could not be depicted

sarcoidosis, amyloidosis, histiocytosis X) [14, 15]. The distinction between a benign dominant stricture and cholangiocarcinoma (CCA) in a PSC patient is challenging (Figs. 8.5, 8.6). As the key cholangiographic features of PSC are annular strictures out of proportion to upstream dilatation due to extended fibrosis, when these ducts are overdilated other sclerosing processes such as ascending cholangitis or CCA on PSC should be considered. In a meta-analysis study [31] MRCP appeared as less reliable for differentiating malignant from benign causes of biliary obstruction than it was for detecting the presence of biliary obstruction in general. This lower accuracy in identifying a malignant cause may be due to its lower spatial resolution and inadequate depiction of the contour of strictures as compared with direct cholangiography (ERCP and PTC). As a matter of fact MRCP reveals only abnormalities in the duct lumen and needs to be combined with parenchymal transverse sections after contrast media administration to detect intra-hepatic CCA [32]. Recognition of typical CCA delayed accumulation and washout of contrast material, due to its fibrous centre, allows a demonstration of

extraductal anomalies suspected for CCA at contrast-enhanced CT or MRI. On MRI, periportal changes, manifesting as low signal intensity on T1w images and high signal intensity on T2w and T1w with late contrast enhancement images, are suggestive of CCA if their extent is greater than 1.5 cm. Cholangiographic features that suggest CCA include irregular high grade ductal narrowing with shouldered margins, rapid progression of the strictures, marked ductal dilatation proximal to strictures and polypoid lesions (Fig. 8.6) [14].

8.2.2 Less Common Bile Duct Disorders in IBD-CU: Variants of PSC

8.2.2.1 Small Duct PSC

A variant of PSC called small duct PSC (sdPSC) is applied to the small percentage of patients with characteristic clinical and biochemical findings of PSC but with a normal cholangiography. The absence of macroscopic abnormalities at MRCP needs a liver biopsy for the diagnosis of sdPSC [8]. This entity was initially

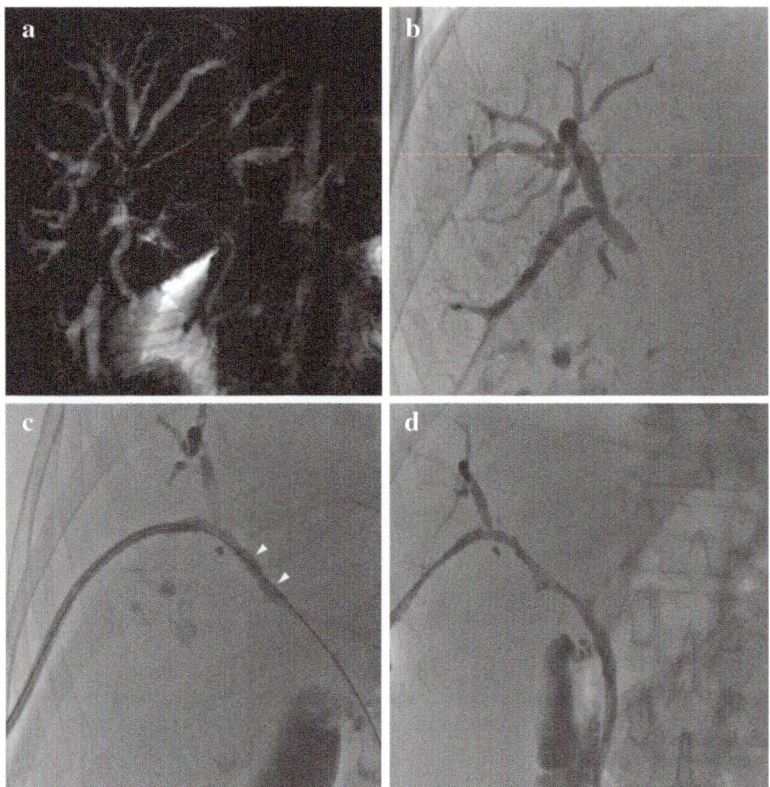

Fig. 8.5 48-year-old male patient with UC and CSP. MRCP **a** shows central stenosis of the biliary tree with marked upstream intra-hepatic ductal dilatation, suspected for CCA. Patient underwent PTC, which confirmed tight stenosis of the *right* main biliary duct (**b**). Bioptic samples excluded neoplasia. After percutaneous balloon dilatation (**c**) and 7 days, drainage resolution of the stenosis and restoration of bile flow were achieved (**d**)

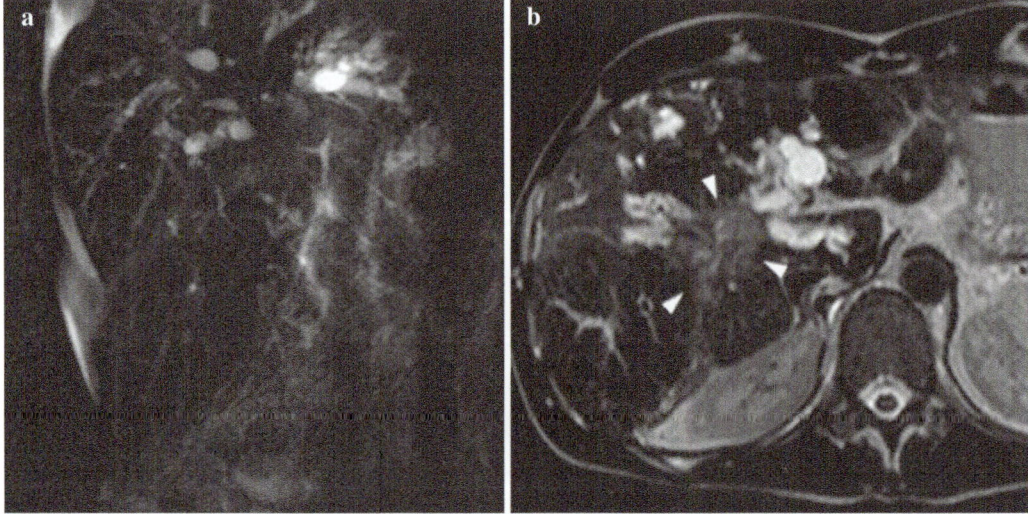

Fig. 8.6 49-year-old male patient with CSP and CCA. MRCP (**a**) shows central stenosis of the biliary tree with marked upstream irregular intra-hepatic ductal dilatation, suspected for CCA. Axial T2w image (**b**) shows 4 cm hilar hyperintense lesion (*arrowheads*) consistent with histologically proven CCA. Note perihepatic fluid collection

termed 'pericholangitis', and includes less than 5 % of PSC cases [15]. SdPSC may be a specific form of HPB disorder associated with IBD and US criteria for the diagnosis mandates the presence of co-existing IBD. In contrast, the presence of IBD was not a part of the criteria to classify sdPSC used in Europe [1]. Unlike the classical form, the presence of IBD does not impact survival in sdPSC [7, 33]. SdPSC appears to have a more favourable prognosis than large duct disease with a median survival of 29.5 years compared to 17 years for classical PSC and CCA has not been described in this variant [3, 7, 15]. Approximately 28 % of patients progress to the large duct variant over a median of 7.4 years [4, 7] which suggests that sdPSC may be an earlier stage of PSC with progression disease to classical PSC and/or end-stage liver disease and consequent need of OLT [3, 34].

8.2.2.2 IgG4-Associated Sclerosing Cholangitis

IgG4-associated cholangitis (IAC) has been proposed as a term to describe the biliary manifestations of the serum immunoglobulin G4-related systemic disease (ISD), which is a steroid responsive multisystem fibro-inflammatory disorder in which affected organs have a characteristic lymphoplasmacytic infiltrate rich in IgG4-positive cells associated with intense sclerosis [15]. Compared with PSC, IAC presents at an older age (mean age, 62 vs. 40 years) and is uncommon in IBD patients (5 %). The systemic fibro-inflammatory process of ISD also involves pancreas, salivary and lacrimal glands, retroperitoneum, kidney and lymph nodes. Thus, other organ involvement is an important clue in the diagnosis of IAC. The association of IAC with autoimmune pancreatitis (AIP) has clinical relevance. Studies from the Mayo Clinic revealed that 92.5 % of patients with IAC suffer from AIP, whereas IAC may occur in 20–90 % of cases of AIP [35]. IAC should be suspected in unexplained biliary strictures associated with increased serum IgG4 and unexplained pancreatic disease [36]. The prevalence of IAC in PSC

patients is reported between 7 and 11.6 % [35]. Nevertheless, IAC appears to be a histologically and pathogenetically distinct entity with dramatic response to corticosteroid therapy in contrast to the progressive and refractory nature of PSC [1]. That is why in all patients with possible PSC, the AASLD guidelines suggest obtaining IgG4 levels to exclude IgG4-associated sclerosing cholangitis [15]. At MRCP and ERCP, IAC is characterized by bile duct wall thickening and biliary strictures, which closely resembles PSC [36].

8.2.2.3 Primary Sclerosing Cholangitis/ Autoimmune Hepatitis (PSC/AIH) Overlap Syndrome

Patients with IBD, especially UC, are also at increased risk of other immune-mediated liver disease including autoimmune hepatitis (AIH). AIH and PSC may also occur within the same individual. It remains unclear if this represents the independent occurrence of both diseases, the presence of a distinct overlap syndrome or different stages in the evolution of a single disease entity [4]. PSC/AIH overlap syndrome is characterized by clinical, biochemical and histological features of autoimmune hepatitis and typical cholangiographic findings of PSC [15]. Typically, patients with IBD develop AIH first and subsequently go on to develop PSC. Patients with PSC/AIH seem to take benefit from treatment with immunosuppressive medications and may have a better prognosis as compared to patients with an isolated PSC [7, 34].

8.3 Liver Involvement

8.3.1 Non-alcoholic Fatty Liver Disease

Fatty changes are commonly seen (from 13 to almost 100 %) in liver biopsy specimens or at US examination in patients with UC [1, 34] and correlate with colitis severity. This contributes a significant proportion of patients with abnormal

LFTs in UC patients. The use of corticosteroids in IBD may be a contributing factor for the development of fatty liver.

8.3.2 Nodular Regenerative Hyperplasia: Medication-Associated Liver Disease

Among HPB manifestation associated with treatment of IBD, nodular regenerative hyperplasia (NRH) has to be taken into consideration. Under thiopurine therapy, 6-thioguanine (6-TG) in particular, in addition to elevated liver enzymes and decreased platelets count, anatomical changes of the liver structure have been described, such as the development of NRH. NRH is considered to be sign of dose-dependent hepatotoxicity of thiopurines, and may ultimately lead to non-cirrhotic portal hypertension with splenomegaly [37, 38]. The outcome of this serious complication consequently influenced the management of patients taking purine analogues suggesting a screen for potential anicteric cholestasis and/or decreased platelet counts and, if positive, performing morphological explorations in order to identify the aetiology [2]. CT and MRI are contributive for diagnosing NRH but a liver biopsy sample may be necessary. NRHs are generally multiple, hypervascularized nodules scattered throughout the liver, with a preferential periportal distribution. Typically, the nodules are bright on unenhanced T1w MR images and enhance strongly following intravenous administration of gadolinium-based contrast agents. On T2w images they are predominantly iso- or hypointense relative to the normal liver. On unenhanced CT scans, NRHs are hyper- or isodense compared with the surrounding liver parenchyma; on MDCT scans, they are markedly and homogeneously hyperattenuating on arterial phase images, they remain slightly hyperattenuating, with peripheral hypodense rim, on portal-venous phase images, and become isodense in the delayed phase. NRH pattern of enhancement can change into a heterogeneous one, with similar features to FNH: hyperdense nodule with central hypodensity and peripheral hypodense rim in the arterial phase and subsequent portal-venous phase, iso- or hypodense with central hyperdense scar in the delayed phase [39].

8.4 Extrahepatic Involvement: Pancreatitis

Patients with UC have an elevated risk for developing pancreatitis as well as pancreatic insufficiency. In the majority of cases, pancreatic involvement is silent and frequency of clinical pancreatitis is lower than that of asymptomatic exocrine pancreas insufficiency [40].

8.4.1 Acute Pancreatitis

Acute pancreatitis can precede, follow or coincide with the occurrence of UC. It is mostly due to medications intake, biliary lithiasis and sclerosing cholangitis. Nevertheless, many cases remain unexplained and are labelled as idiopathic pancreatitis, in which autoimmune mechanisms are believed to play a major role [41]. Acute pancreatitis is commonly reported with 6-Mercaptopurine (6-MP) and Azathioprine (AZA), used in IBD treatment. It is an early idiosyncratic and dose-independent adverse reaction after initiation of treatment, occurring within 3–4 weeks of therapy and disappearing in 1–11 days after withdrawing the drug. In patients with PSC, both bile and pancreatic ducts can be affected by the same autoimmune process resulting in an acute "sclerosing pancreatitis" [42]. Imaging plays a major role in the evaluation of acute pancreatitis, confirming the clinical diagnosis, depicting its cause and grading its extent and severity. Cross-sectional imaging allows exclusion of alternative causes of abdominal pain and early detection of complications, such as necrosis, pseudocyst, pseudoaneurysm and abscesses. Contrast-enhanced CT is the imaging modality of choice for evaluating acute pancreatitis. Pancreas may appear either normal-sized or enlarged with sharp margins and a variable amount of peripancreatic fat "stranding", which consist of exudate, fat tissue necrosis or haemorrhage. CT is 100 % specific for necrosis, defined by a not enhanced 30 % of the gland, developing between 24 and 48 h after the onset of acute pancreatitis. MRI is comparable with CT. T2w sequences are particularly useful for the detection of peripancreatic collections and the evaluation of the main pancreatic duct, which is often dilated. MRCP is not recommended for identifying the cause of acute pancreatitis, because collections may compress pancreatic and biliary ducts obscuring gallstones [43].

8.4.2 Autoimmune Pancreatitis

Autoimmune pancreatitis (AIP) is currently considered to represent the pancreatic manifestation of IgG4-related systemic disease, in which affected organs show dense lymphoplasmacytic infiltration with abundant IgG4-positive cells. It is known that in patients with AIP prevalence of IBD is higher than that in the general population [40–44]. Patients typically present with jaundice or abdominal discomfort; severe abdominal pain or acute pancreatitis is unusual. Affected areas typically appear hypoechoic at US, hypoattenuating at CT, mildly hyperintense at T2w and hypointense on T1w fat-suppressed MRI images. Common pancreatic duct is narrowed and irregular. There are three patterns of AIP: diffuse, focal and multifocal. Diffuse disease, the most common, consists in a whole pancreas enlargement, with sharp margin and loss of the lobular contour. Focal disease can mimic a pancreatic malignancy: it manifests as a focal mass often involving the pancreatic head and causing upstream dilatation of the main pancreatic duct. Unlike pancreatic carcinoma, focal AIP is well demarcated and pancreatic duct dilatation is mild. Involvement of the pancreatic head can cause narrowing of the intrapancreatic portion of the common bile duct. Features that suggest the diagnosis of autoimmune pancreatitis over acute pancreatitis include minimal or no peripancreatic stranding and the presence of a capsule-like rim or "halo" representing

peripancreatic oedema or fibrous tissue; furthermore, pancreatic function and morphologic characteristics usually return to normal within 4–6 weeks of corticosteroid therapy [45].

8.4.3 Chronic Pancreatitis

IBD-associated chronic pancreatitis predominantly occurs in an asymptomatic form. Symptoms of chronic pancreatitis were found in only 2 % of patients, while autopsy series on patients with IBD showed histologic signs of pancreatitis in 38–53 %. It has been suggested that epithelial cells of gastrointestinal and pancreatic tissue may share similar target molecular or cellular structures [46]. MR is the mainstay imaging modality in the assessment of chronic pancreatitis: it allows an accurate evaluation of both parenchymal and ductal changes on static images and during hormonal stimulation. Patients with clinically diagnosed chronic pancreatitis should undergo MRCP to evaluate ductal changes and obstructive causes of chronic pancreatitis (biliary lithiasis) together with contrast-enhanced MR of the pancreas to evaluate parenchymal signal changes and gland perfusion. Dynamic secretin-stimulated MRCP demonstrates ductal changes due to parenchymal fibrosis, related to severity of the disease, and estimates exocrine function by grading duodenal filling. Diffusion-weighted imaging (DWI) is an emerging technique that could have a role in quantifying parenchymal response to secretin stimulation [47].

References

1. Navaneethan U, Shen B (2010) Hepatopancreatobiliary manifestations and complications associated with inflammatory bowel disease. Inflamm Bowel Dis 16:1598–1619
2. Nahon S, Cadranel JF, Chazouilleres O et al (2009) Liver and inflammatory bowel disease. Gastroenterol Clin Biol 33:370–381
3. Angulo P, Maor-Kendler Y, Lindor KD (2002) Small-duct primary sclerosing cholangitis: a long-term follow-up study. Hepatology 35:1494–1500
4. Saich R, Chapman R (2008) Primary sclerosing cholangitis, autoimmune hepatitis and overlap

syndromes in inflammatory bowel disease. World J Gastroenterol 14:331–337

5. Bambha K, Kim WR, Talwalkar J et al (2003) Incidence, clinical spectrum, and outcomes of primary sclerosing cholangitis in a United States community. Gastroenterology 125:1364–1369

6. Smith MP, Loe RH (1965) Sclerosing cholangitis; review of recent case reports and associated diseases and four new cases. Am J Surg 110:239–246

7. Trivedi PJ, Chapman RW (2012) PSC, AIH and overlap syndrome in inflammatory bowel disease. Clin Res Hepatol Gastroenterol 36:420–436

8. Van Assche G, Dignass A, Bokemeyer B et al (2013) Second European evidence-based consensus on the diagnosis and management of ulcerative colitis part 3: Special situations. J Crohns Colitis 7:1–33

9. Loftus EV Jr, Harewood GC, Loftus CG et al (2005) PSC-IBD: a unique form of inflammatory bowel disease associated with primary sclerosing cholangitis. Gut 54:91–96

10. Biancone L, Michetti P, Travis S et al (2008) European evidence-based consensus on the management of ulcerative colitis: special situations. J Crohns Colitis 2:63–92

11. Dignass A, Eliakim R, Magro F et al (2012) Second European evidence-based consensus on the diagnosis and management of ulcerative colitis part 1: definitions and diagnosis. J Crohns Colitis 6:965–990

12. Rabinovitz M, Gavaler JS, Schade RR et al (1990) Does primary sclerosing cholangitis occurring in association with inflammatory bowel disease differ from that occurring in the absence of inflammatory bowel disease? A study of sixty-six subjects. Hepatology 11:7–11

13. Chapman RW, Jewell DP (1985) Primary sclerosing cholangitis–an immunologically mediated disease? West J Med 143:193–195

14. Vitellas KM, Keogan MT, Freed KS et al (2000) Radiologic manifestations of sclerosing cholangitis with emphasis on MR cholangiopancreatography. Radiographics 20:959–975; quiz 1108–1109, 1112

15. Lichtenstein DR (2011) Hepatobiliary complications of inflammatory bowel disease. Curr Gastroenterol Rep 13:495–505

16. Chapman R, Fevery J, Kalloo A et al (2010) Diagnosis and management of primary sclerosing cholangitis. Hepatology 51:660–678

17. Broome U, Lofberg R, Veress B, Eriksson LS (1995) Primary sclerosing cholangitis and ulcerative colitis: evidence for increased neoplastic potential. Hepatology 22:1404–1408

18. Enns R (2008) The use of ERCP versus MRCP in primary sclerosing cholangitis. Gastroenterol Hepatol (NY) 4:852–854

19. MacCarty RL, LaRusso NF, Wiesner RH, Ludwig J (1983) Primary sclerosing cholangitis: findings on cholangiography and pancreatography. Radiology 149:39–44

20. Panes J, Bouhnik Y, Reinisch W et al (2013) Imaging techniques for assessment of inflammatory bowel disease: joint ECCO and ESGAR evidence-based consensus guidelines. J Crohns Colitis 7(7):556–585

21. Fulcher AS, Turner MA, Franklin KJ et al (2000) Primary sclerosing cholangitis: evaluation with MR cholangiography-a case-control study. Radiology 215:71–80

22. Cohen SA, Siegel JH, Kasmin FE (1996) Complications of diagnostic and therapeutic ERCP. Abdom Imaging 21:385–394

23. Dave M, Elmunzer BJ, Dwamena BA, Higgins PD (2010) Primary sclerosing cholangitis: meta-analysis of diagnostic performance of MR cholangiopancreatography. Radiology 256:387–396

24. Aljiffry M, Renfrew PD, Walsh MJ, Laryea M, Molinari M (2011) Analytical review of diagnosis and treatment strategies for dominant bile duct strictures in patients with primary sclerosing cholangitis. HPB (Oxford) 13:79–90

25. Fulcher AS (2004) Magnetic resonance cholangiopancreatography: is it becoming the study of choice for evaluating obstructive jaundice? J Clin Gastroenterol 38:839–840

26. Moff SL, Kamel IR, Eustace J et al (2006) Diagnosis of primary sclerosing cholangitis: a blinded comparative study using magnetic resonance cholangiography and endoscopic retrograde cholangiography. Gastrointest Endosc 64:219–223

27. Dusunceli E, Erden A, Erden I, Karayalcin S (2005) Primary sclerosing cholangitis: MR cholangiopancreatography and T2-weighted MR imaging findings. Diagn Interv Radiol 11:213–218

28. Ernst O, Asselah T, Sergent G et al (1998) MR cholangiography in primary sclerosing cholangitis. Am J Roentgenol 171:1027–1030

29. Berstad AE, Aabakken L, Smith HJ et al (2006) Diagnostic accuracy of magnetic resonance and endoscopic retrograde cholangiography in primary sclerosing cholangitis. Clin Gastroenterol Hepatol 4:514–520

30. Vitellas KM, El-Dieb A, Vaswani KK et al (2002) MR cholangiopancreatography in patients with primary sclerosing cholangitis: interobserver variability and comparison with endoscopic retrograde cholangiopancreatography. Am J Roentgenol 179:399–407

31. Romagnuolo J, Bardou M, Rahme E et al (2003) Magnetic resonance cholangiopancreatography: a meta-analysis of test performance in suspected biliary disease. Ann Intern Med 139:547–557

32. Revelon G, Rashid A, Kawamoto S, Bluemke DA (1999) Primary sclerosing cholangitis: MR imaging findings with pathologic correlation. Am J Roentgenol 173:1037–1042

33. Charatcharoenwitthaya P, Angulo P, Enders FB, Lindor KD (2008) Impact of inflammatory bowel disease and ursodeoxycholic acid therapy on small-duct primary sclerosing cholangitis. Hepatology 47:133–142

34. Uko V, Thangada S, Radhakrishnan K (2012) Liver disorders in inflammatory bowel disease. Gastroenterol Res Pract 2012:642923

35. Parhizkar B, Mohammad Alizadeh AH, Asadzadeh Aghdaee H, Malekpour H, Entezari AH (2012) Primary sclerosing cholangitis associated with elevated immunoglobulin-g4: a preliminary study. ISRN Gastroenterol 2012:325743
36. Ghazale A, Chari ST, Zhang L et al (2008) Immunoglobulin G4-associated cholangitis: clinical profile and response to therapy. Gastroenterology 134:706–715
37. Ferlitsch A, Teml A, Reinisch W et al (2007) 6-thioguanine associated nodular regenerative hyperplasia in patients with inflammatory bowel disease may induce portal hypertension. Am J Gastroenterol 102:2495–2503
38. Rogler G (2010) Gastrointestinal and liver adverse effects of drugs used for treating IBD. Best Pract Res Clin Gastroenterol 24:157–165
39. Flor N, Zuin M, Brovelli F et al (2010) Regenerative nodules in patients with chronic Budd-Chiari syndrome: a longitudinal study using multiphase contrast-enhanced multidetector CT. Eur J Radiol 73:588–593
40. Barthet M, Lesavre N, Desplats S et al (2006) Frequency and characteristics of pancreatitis in patients with inflammatory bowel disease. Pancreatology 6:464–471
41. Saez J, Martinez J, Garcia C, Grino P, Perez-Mateo M (2000) Idiopathic pancreatitis associated with ulcerative colitis. Am J Gastroenterol 95:3004–3005
42. Inoue H, Shiraki K, Okano H et al (2005) Acute pancreatitis in patients with ulcerative colitis. Dig Dis Sci 50:1064–1067
43. O'Connor OJ, McWilliams S, Maher MM (2011) Imaging of acute pancreatitis. Am J Roentgenol 197:W221–W225
44. Ghazale AH, Chari ST, Vege SS (2008) Update on the diagnosis and treatment of autoimmune pancreatitis. Curr Gastroenterol Rep 10:115–121
45. Vlachou PA, Khalili K, Jang HJ et al (2011) IgG4-related sclerosing disease: autoimmune pancreatitis and extrapancreatic manifestations. Radiographics 31:1379–1402
46. Barthet M, Hastier P, Bernard JP et al (1999) Chronic pancreatitis and inflammatory bowel disease: true or coincidental association? Am J Gastroenterol 94:2141–2148
47. Balci C (2011) MRI assessment of chronic pancreatitis. Diagn Interv Radiol 17:249–254

Vascular Complications of Ulcerative Colitis

Massimo Tonolini

Individuals affected with chronic inflammatory bowel diseases (IBD) have a potential hypercoagulable state, and an increased risk of developing thromboembolic events compared to the general population. Overall, in IBD patients, venous thrombosis is reported with a 1–8 % prevalence in clinical series, in up to 41 % of cases in autopsy series, and particularly during perioperative hospitalization [1–4].

In patients with Ulcerative Colitis (UC), the risk of thrombosis is approximately doubled compared with controls. Venous thromboembolism that is reported in 1.2–6.7 % patients in the largest series most usually occurs during active UC phases and represents a significant cause of UC-related morbidity and mortality. Lower limbs deep vein thrombosis and pulmonary embolism are the most common clinical manifestations, whereas in rare instances the cerebral and retinal veins may be affected [5].

Although relatively rare, portal venous system thrombosis (PVT) is increasingly recognized as a serious extraintestinal complication of UC with an estimated 0.1–1 % overall prevalence. The most relevant risk factors include active bowel inflammation, post-operative status and cigarette smoking. The complex, multifactorial pathogenesis of PVT associates regional causes such as abdominal sepsis and recent surgical manipulation of abdominal veins, with systemic abnormalities such as chronic hypercoagulability and thrombocytosis, and acquired factors such as smoking, oral contraception use and prolonged bed rest [3, 4, 6].

Although it may develop during either acute phases or clinical remission, PVT is most usually observed during exacerbations or shortly after surgery. Post-operatively, the incidence of PVT has been reported to reach 5 % of patients following restorative proctocolectomy [1–4, 6, 7].

Clinical manifestations of PVT are usually subtle and non-specific and include abdominal pain or discomfort, fever, abnormal laboratory acute phase reactants and liver enzymes, sometimes positive hemocultures. Abnormal liver laboratory tests are commonly encountered in patients with UC, and may be secondary to intrinsic disease manifestations, or otherwise attributed to treatments. Among the spectrum of possible underlying causes, the most usual conditions include sclerosing cholangitis (which is discussed in depth in Chap. 8 of this book), hepatic steatosis, gallstone disease and drug toxicity [4, 6]. Not unusually, PVT may be incidentally detected in asymptomatic patients. Therefore, both clinicians and radiologists should maintain a high level of suspicion not to miss this important diagnosis [2, 8].

Unrecognized PVT may lead to long-term development of cavernomatous transformation, portal biliopathy or portal hypertension, and to possible life-threatening complications such as

M. Tonolini (✉)
Radiology Department, "Luigi Sacco" University Hospital, Via G.B. Grassi 74, 20157 Milan, Italy
e-mail: mtonolini@sirm.org

M. Tonolini (ed.), *Imaging of Ulcerative Colitis*,
DOI: 10.1007/978-88-470-5409-7_9, © Springer-Verlag Italia 2014

bleeding esophageal varices and splenic rupture. Although not standardized, conservative treatment with intravenous broad-spectrum antibiotics coupled with heparin or oral anticoagulation usually cures PVT [4, 7]. Invasive thrombolytic therapies such as transhepatic intraportal infusion of plasminogen activators have been attempted in refractory cases [9].

Contrast-enhanced multidetector CT including a full venous phase acquisition allows comprehensive visualization of the spleno-portal-mesenteric venous system and the detection of intravascular opacification defects consistent with thrombosis, not unusually involving multiple sites (Figs. 9.1, 9.2). Radiologists should be aware of the possibility of PVT when imaging

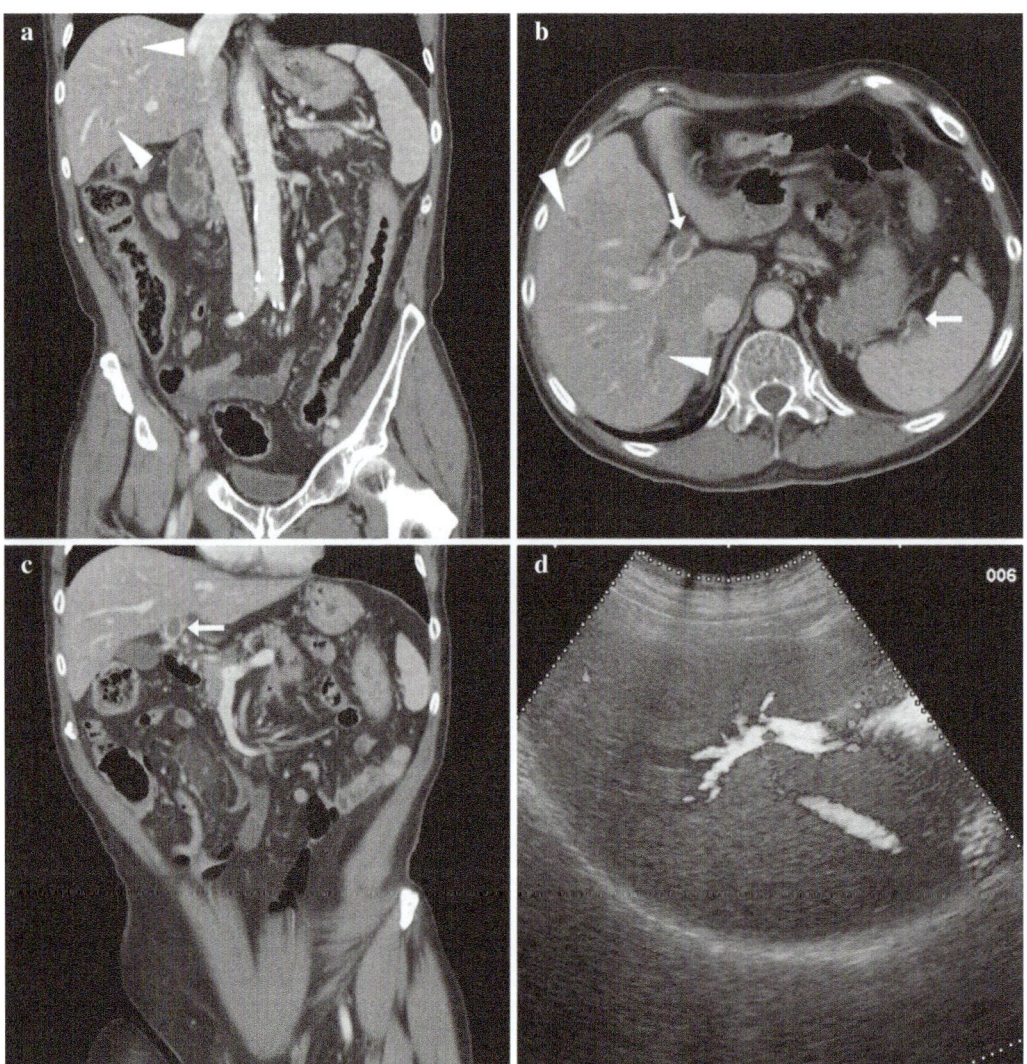

Fig. 9.1 22-year-old male patient affected with medically treated extensive Ulcerative Colitis (UC), hospitalized during a febrile disease exacerbation. Contrast-enhanced multidetector CT (MDCT) shows enhancing mural thickening corresponding to clinical and endoscopic active UC throughout the *left* colon (**a**). Additionally, opacification defects corresponding to partial thrombosis are seen in multiple intrahepatic portal vein branches (*arrows*), and in the portal trunk and distal splenic vein (*arrowheads*), whereas the mesenteric vein is patent (**b, c**). Following antibiotic and anticoagulant therapy, colour Doppler ultrasound detected patency of the portal vein (**d**). Subsequently, restorative proctocolectomy was performed

patients with UC, particularly during acute exacerbations or in the early post-operative period, and carefully scrutinize the spleno-porto-mesenteric venous system to identify subtle thromboses [10–12].

Ultrasound may non-invasively detect gross thrombosis in an enlarged portal vein with echogenic lumen and absent colour Doppler flow signal. However, in comparison to CT, ultrasound lacks panoramicity and the ability to assess small intrahepatic portal branches. Therefore, colour Doppler ultrasound may be helpful to initially detect extensive thrombosis, or to follow-up treated PVT in order to limit irradiation from repeated CT studies (Figs. 9.1, 9.2) [13].

Proctocolectomy has been reported to cure PVT. Following proctocolectomy in UC patients, CT is frequently requested (in up to 25 % of

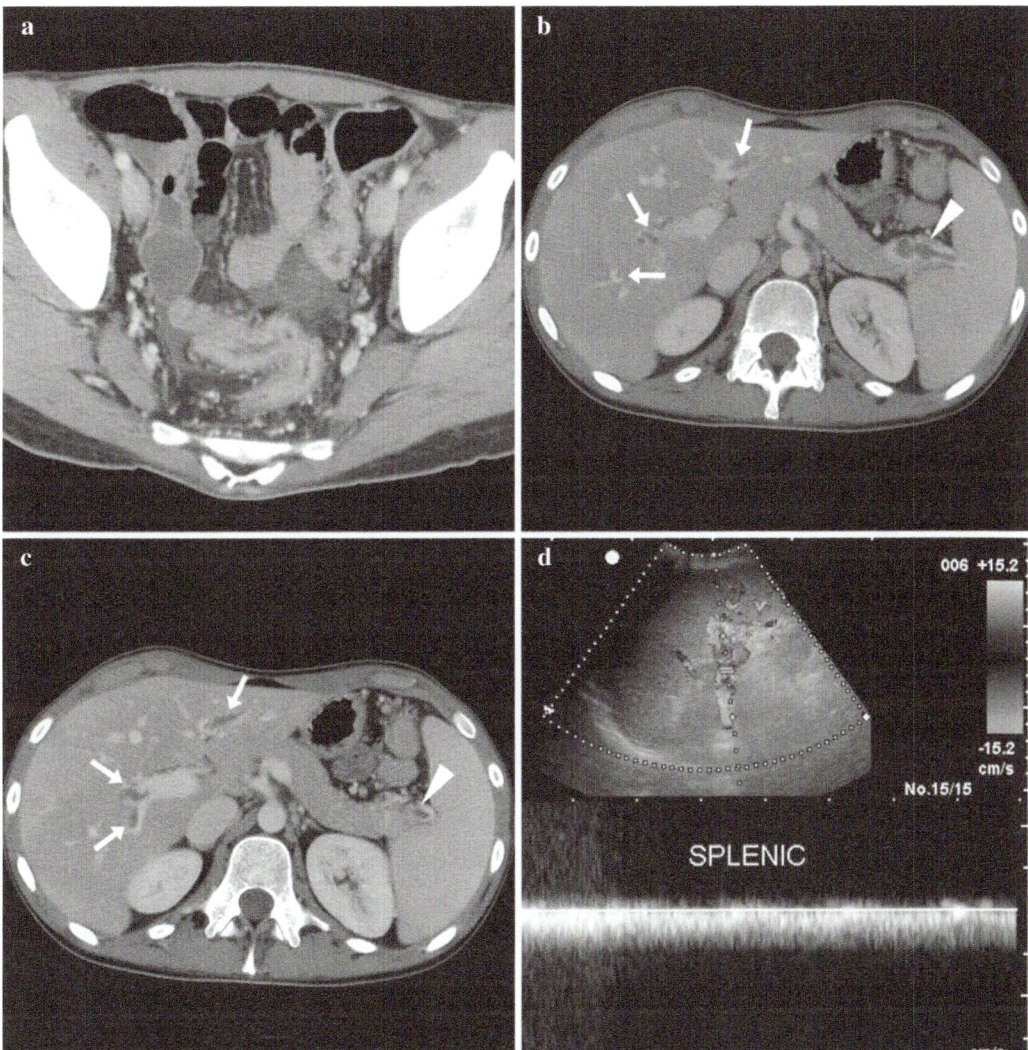

Fig. 9.2 66-year-old male patient with UC, without previous surgical treatment, investigated during an acute exacerbation. Axial contrast-enhanced MDCT images show inflammatory sigmoiditis and minimal ascites in (**a**). As an unexpected finding (**b, c**) extensive thrombosis of the splenic vein (*arrowhead*) and multiple partial thromboses of the intrahepatic portal branches (*arrows*) are identified. After treatment, colour Doppler ultrasound (**d**) shows reappearance of normal flow in the patent splenic vein

operated patients) during the post-operative
hospital stay to investigate clinical complaints
(such as persistent pain and/or fever, ascites or
prolonged ileus) or laboratory abnormalities, and
to rule out possible complications. Retrospective
studies detected PVT in as much as 39–45 %

of those post-operative patients who were
investigated with CT (Fig. 9.3). Interestingly, a
significant proportion of thromboses had
been missed during initial interpretation of
post-operative CT examinations. Furthermore,
pre-operative presence of PVT is associated with

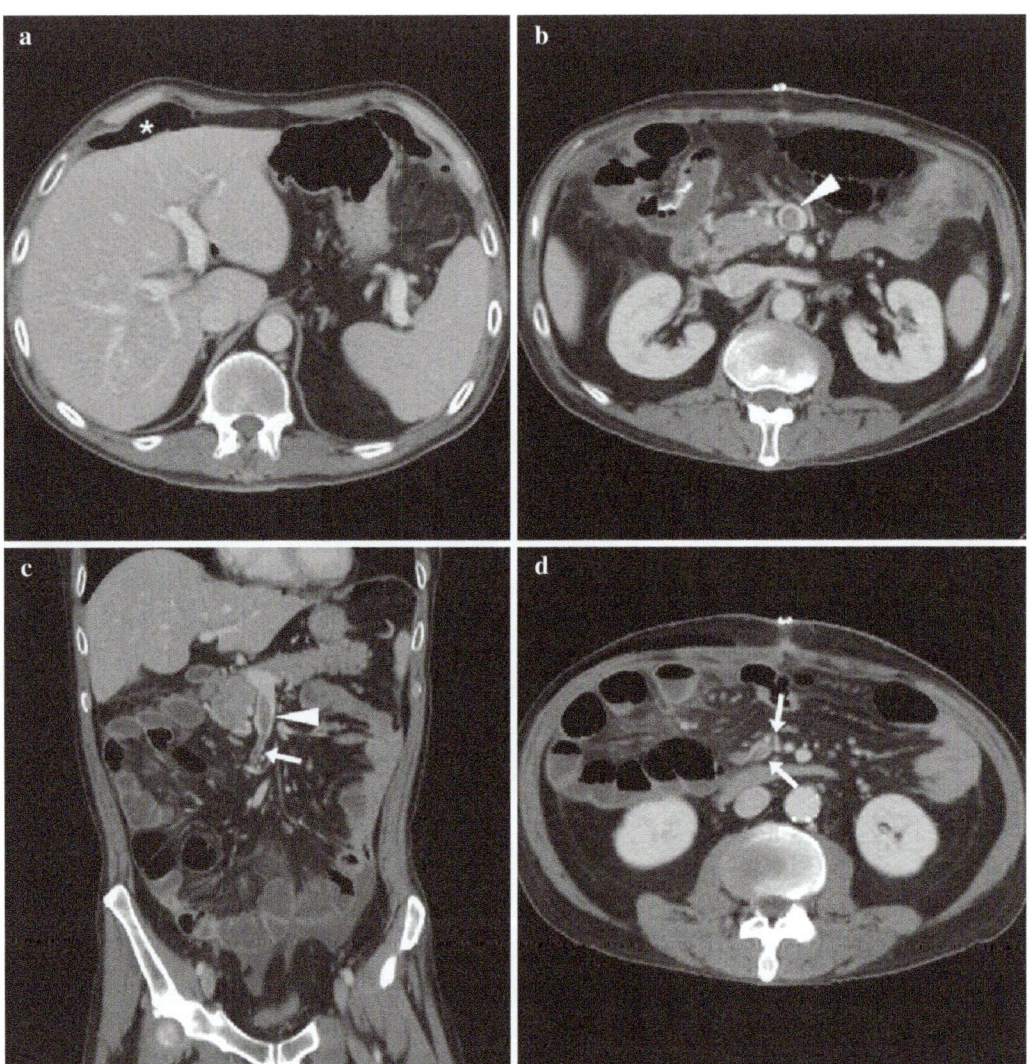

Fig. 9.3 40-year-old male patient with UC, seven days
after proctocolectomy surgery. Axial contrast-enhanced
MDCT images (**a**, **b**) show post-surgical condition with
minimal residual air (*) in the peritoneal cavity, and a
subtotal opacification defect (*arrowhead* in **b**) consistent
with thrombosis of the superior mesenteric vein. Coronal
reformatted (**c**) and distal axial (**d**) images depict the
longitudinal extent of the mesenteric thrombosis (*arrowhead* in **c**) and the involvement of at least two branches
(*arrows*)

an estimated 45 % risk for subsequent pouchitis compared with 15.4 % for patients without PVT [3, 8, 10, 11].

References

1. Fichera A, Cicchiello LA, Mendelson DS et al (2003) Superior mesenteric vein thrombosis after colectomy for inflammatory bowel disease: a not uncommon cause of postoperative acute abdominal pain. Dis Colon Rectum 46:643–648
2. Hatoum OA, Spinelli KS, Abu-Hajir M et al (2005) Mesenteric venous thrombosis in inflammatory bowel disease. J Clin Gastroenterol 39:27–31
3. Jackson CS, Fryer J, Danese S et al (2011) Mesenteric vascular thromboembolism in inflammatory bowel disease: a single center experience. J Gastrointest Surg 15:97–100
4. Navaneethan U, Shen B (2010) Hepatopancreatobiliary manifestations and complications associated with inflammatory bowel disease. Inflamm Bowel Dis 16:1598–1619
5. Van Assche G, Dignass A, Bokemeyer B et al (2013) Second European evidence-based consensus on the diagnosis and management of ulcerative colitis part 3: special situations. J Crohns Colitis 7:1–33
6. Nahon S, Cadranel JF, Chazouilleres O et al (2009) Liver and inflammatory bowel disease. Gastroenterol Clin Biol 33:370–381
7. Mijnhout GS, Klinkenberg EC, Lycklama G et al (2004) Sepsis and elevated liver enzymes in a patient with inflammatory bowel disease: think of portal vein thrombosis. Dig Liver Dis 36:296–300
8. Millan M, Hull TL, Hammel J et al (2007) Portal vein thrombi after restorative proctocolectomy: serious complication without long-term sequelae. Dis Colon Rectum 50:1540–1544
9. Guglielmi A, Fior F, Halmos O et al (2005) Transhepatic fibrinolysis of mesenteric and portal vein thrombosis in a patient with ulcerative colitis: a case report. World J Gastroenterol 11:2035–2038
10. Remzi FH, Fazio VW, Oncel M et al. (2002) Portal vein thrombi after restorative proctocolectomy. Surgery 132:655–661 (discussion 661–652)
11. Ball CG, MacLean AR, Buie WD et al (2007) Portal vein thrombi after ileal pouch-anal anastomosis: its incidence and association with pouchitis. Surg Today 37:552–557
12. Lefevre A, Soyer P, Vahedi K et al (2011) Multiple intra-abdominal venous thrombosis in ulcerative colitis: role of MDCT for detection. Clin Imaging 35:68–72
13. Maconi G, Bolzacchini E, Dell'era A et al (2012) Portal vein thrombosis in inflammatory bowel diseases: a single-center case series. J Crohns Colitis 6:362–367

Neoplasms in Ulcerative Colitis

10

Massimo Tonolini

10.1 Colorectal Cancer Detection and Staging

It is widely known that individuals affected with chronic inflammatory bowel diseases (IBD) have an increased risk of intestinal cancer compared to the general population. Although only 1 % of all cases of colorectal carcinoma (CRC) occur in patients with Ulcerative Colitis (UC) , IBD represent one of the highest risk groups for developing CRC. In the longest prospectively collected database on UC surveillance, the cumulative cancer incidence has been estimated at 2.5 % at 20 years, 7.6 % after 30 years and 10.8 % at 40 years. Several other studies reported incidences ranging from 2.1 to 7.5 % [1–4].

In UC, the risk of developing CRC is associated with the cumulative effect of chronic inflammation, and depends on a combination of disease duration, extent of colonic involvement and degree of inflammation severity. Patients with the highest risk are those with early onset (age below 20 at diagnosis) long-standing UC. Concerning disease extent, the risk is highest in extensive colitis, intermediate in patients with left-sided colitis and not increased in proctitis. Several studies have confirmed that the histological severity of inflammation on biopsies independently predicts risk of CRC. Additionally, positive family history of CRC independent of IBD and co-existent primary sclerosing cholangitis (PSC) may further contribute to the individual patient's risk, suggesting the role of an underlying genetic predisposition [1, 2, 4–6].

Molecular biology studies report that the key molecular changes found in sporadic CRC contribute to colitis-associated CRC too, but the timing and sequence in which gene mutations occur differ from sporadic CRC. Whereas APC loss is usually considered an early stage in the adenoma-carcinoma sequence, and p53 represents the final mutation that gives rise to carcinoma, the opposite is true in IBD-associated CRC. Furthermore, in UC carcinoma may develop without any apparent preceding dysplastic change, and low-grade dysplasia may regress or turn into CRC without evolving through high-grade dysplasia [1].

The current clinical guidelines advocate periodic optical colonoscopy (OC) as the cornerstone of prevention. Surveillance programmes have been developed and should be followed to provide earlier detection of dysplastic changes and CRC, reduced CRC-related morbidity and mortality and therefore an improved prognosis. An initial screening OC should be scheduled 6–8 years after the beginning of symptoms, in order to assess the patient's individual risk profile. With left-sided or extensive UC, high-risk patients including those with endoscopic and histological extensive

M. Tonolini (✉)
Radiology Department, "Luigi Sacco" University Hospital, Via G.B. Grassi 74, 20157 Milan, Italy
e-mail: mtonolini@sirm.org

M. Tonolini (ed.), *Imaging of Ulcerative Colitis*,
DOI: 10.1007/978-88-470-5409-7_10, © Springer-Verlag Italia 2014

and/or severe disease, and those with concurrent PSC, should receive colonoscopy every 1–2 years. Conversely, low-risk patients should have OC scheduled every 3–4 years [1, 2, 4].

Tumours are most frequently found in the left-sided large bowel, reflecting the prevalent distribution of UC disease. When dysplasia or early carcinomas are detected, proctocolectomy is indicated as a potentially curative procedure for both cancer and colitis [1, 2, 4, 7].

Unfortunately, conventional OC is less sensitive for detecting precancerous changes in UC than in the general population. In fact, dysplasia in IBD is often found in flat areas that are indistinct from the surrounding diseased mucosa, and therefore missed by the endoscopist. Recently, novel techniques such as magnification colonoscopy, chromoendoscopy, narrow band imaging, autofluorescence and confocal endomicroscopy are increasingly employed to overcome limitations of white-light OC and multisite biopsies, with the goal to improve the detection of dysplasia, and ultimately to increase the yield of CRC surveillance [8–10].

However, failure in early detection of CRC may still occur in UC patients, because of poor adherence to surveillance programmes, of occurrence in strictured areas which cannot be explored by OC, or because IBD-related CRC may develop as a flat lesion [11].

Although intestinal obstruction is most usually due to benign IBD-related complications, the diagnosis of CRC should be considered in long-standing UC patients, particularly without adequate endoscopic surveillance, when symptoms develop after a long period of quiescent disease, or with signs of bowel obstruction [11].

The endoscopic detection of a colonic stenosis in UC should raise the suspicion of CRC, so that multiple biopsies and additional imaging are necessary. In the past, investigation of the mucosal pattern of a stricture, and of proximal upstream colitis was performed by means of double contrast barium enema. Currently, multidetector CT (MDCT) is usually requested to investigate UC patients with suspicious endoscopic changes, detection of colonic neoplasms or stricture [5, 6, 11, 12].

As extensively discussed elsewhere in this book, cross-sectional imaging currently plays a valuable role in the assessment of extent and severity of UC, and of its possible complications, with MDCT acting as the cornerstone modality. Therefore, the role of the radiologist may be crucial in both alerting the referring gastroenterologist when suspected imaging changes are observed in a patient with colitis, or to stage endoscopically detected CRC [11].

A very recent study addressed the imaging features of neoplasms arising in IBD that did not show specific differences between UC and Crohn's disease-related cases. In a cohort of 17 cases, CRC was indiscernible on MDCT from the underlying IBD in at least half of patients (53 %), and visible in the remaining 47 %. The two main reasons for the limited sensitivity are that CRC often develops in colorectal segments involved by IBD, with diffuse mural thickening, distortion and luminal narrowing and that IBD-related CRC is often flat, in agreement with the limited sensitivity of OC (59 %) [11].

Approximately half of MDCT-visible CRCs manifested as a colorectal soft-tissue mass with a 3.5 cm median size, intra- and/or extraluminal growth; extraluminal growth was only noted in two rectal tumours. Alternatively, CRC appears as a circumferential mural thickening, usually severe (over 15 mm), with loss of mural stratification, and heterogeneous enhancement. These features should be viewed with strong suspicion particularly when associated with upstream dilatation indicating luminal obstruction. Additionally, a diagnosis of cancer may be suggested by the detection of adenopathies, liver metastases, peritoneal nodules or effusion [11].

Water enema multidetector CT colonography (WE-MDCT), performed with the same protocol described in Chap. 4 of this book, is considered as the preferred imaging technique in patients with suspected or proven CRC, as it provides excellent visualization of the enhanced bowel wall, and good contrast to the hypodense lumen and pericolonic fat. WE-MDCT is a reliable technique to detect and comprehensively stage CRC, which has significant advantages compared to air or CO_2 CT colonography including optimal patient tolerance, short learning curve without need for complex post processing, pre-surgical multiplanar visualization with submillimetre spatial resolution, high accuracy for assessment of both mural colonic diseases and associated extramural findings [13–15]. Furthermore, WE-MDCT detects CRC in patients with incomplete colonoscopy because of a distal narrowing, even with limited or no preparation, and obviates the risk of perforation with air colon distension, which is highest in IBD patients because of the inflamed, more fragile intestinal wall [13, 15, 16].

In the general population, WE-MDCT has shown a 100 % overall sensitivity, specificity, positive and negative predictive value for the

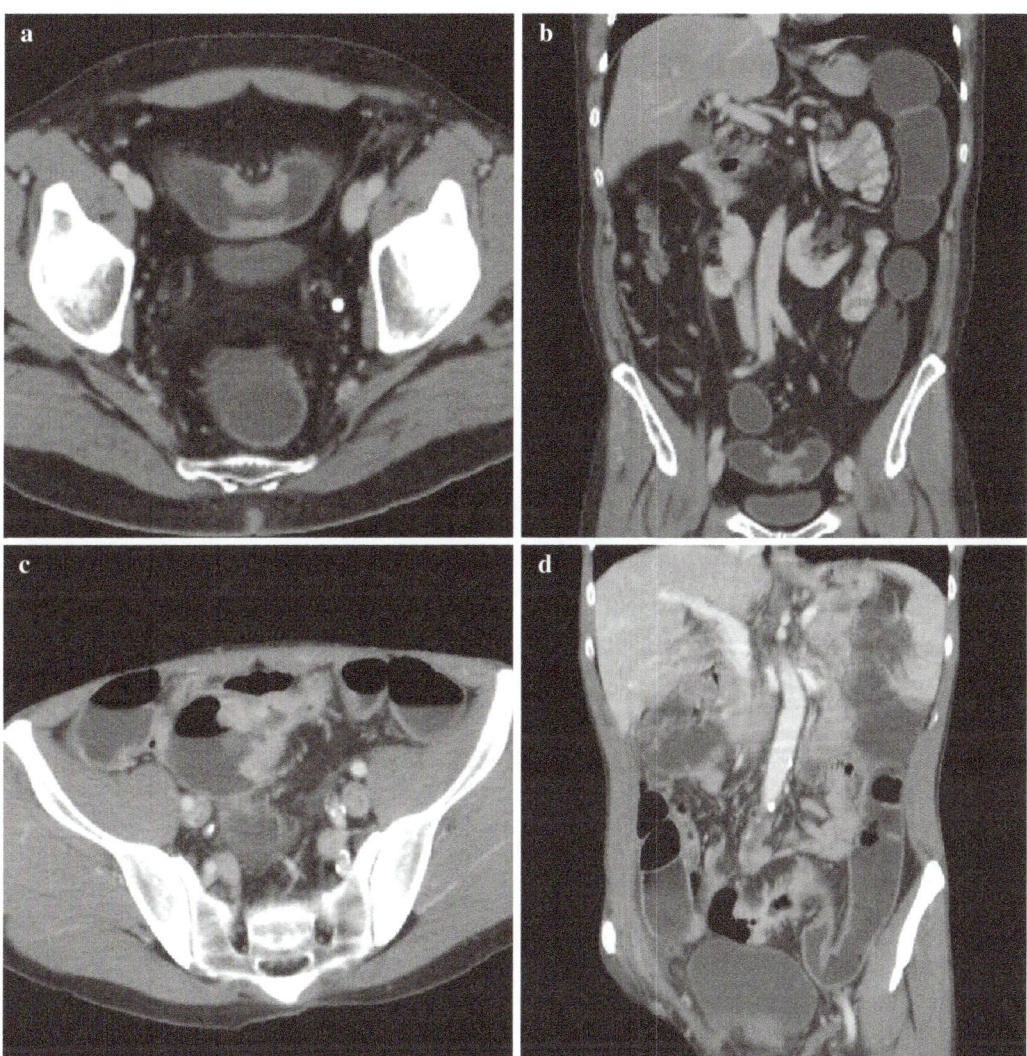

Fig. 10.1 59-year-old male patient with endoscopically detected sigmoid colon carcinoma. Water enema multidetector CT (**a**, **b**) depicts a 5-cm long lesion with circumferential mural thickening and regular external borders, consistent with a T2 stage tumour. In another 52-year-old male patient with an endoscopically impassable stage sigmoid colon cancer, an enhancing mural thickening with pericolonic fat infiltration (T3 stage) and luminal stenosis is detected (**c**, **d**). In both cases water enema CT colonography allows comprehensive exploration of the upstream colon, nodal and visceral staging

detection of colonic neoplasms on a per-patient basis. Per-lesion sensitivity is 87 % overall, 96 % for lesions greater or equal to 6 mm, 99 % for lesions greater or equal to 1 cm and 100 % for malignant lesions [14, 17]. In another study, in patients with clinically suspected CRC, WE-MDCT proved a 98.6 % per-patient sensitivity and 95 % specificity compared to colonoscopy and surgical findings, with 92.1 % positive and 99.1 % predictive values [13, 15].

The key limitation of all radiologic techniques is the detection of flat lesions. At CT, the presence of a neoplasm is defined as a local thickening of the colonic wall measuring at least 1 cm, with irregular edges and heterogeneous enhancement (Fig. 10.1). WE-MDCT allows measurement of lesions' length and thickness, definition of their location along the bowel, detection of pericolonic fat infiltration, lymph-adenopathies, liver metastases, other

extracolonic abnormalities and peritoneal carcinomatosis. According to the usual staging criteria, a T1/T2 tumour has smooth, intact external edges, whereas T3 lesions show irregular edges or frank invasion of pericolic fat. T4 stage is defined by the identification of adjacent organ infiltration. Concerning the definition of the local T stage, WE-MDCT proved to be more accurate (88.6 %) than air CT colonography (80 %), whereas similar accuracy rates (77.1 % vs. 74.3 %) were reported concerning nodal (N) staging [13, 15, 18].

Alternatively, tumours of the rectum are exquisitely visualized by means of external phased-array coils Magnetic Resonance Imaging (MRI) as solid rectal wall thickening with abnormal signal intensity and enhancement (Fig. 10.2). MRI comprehensively demonstrates the tumour height and size, its extramural growth, the presence of perirectal lymph nodes

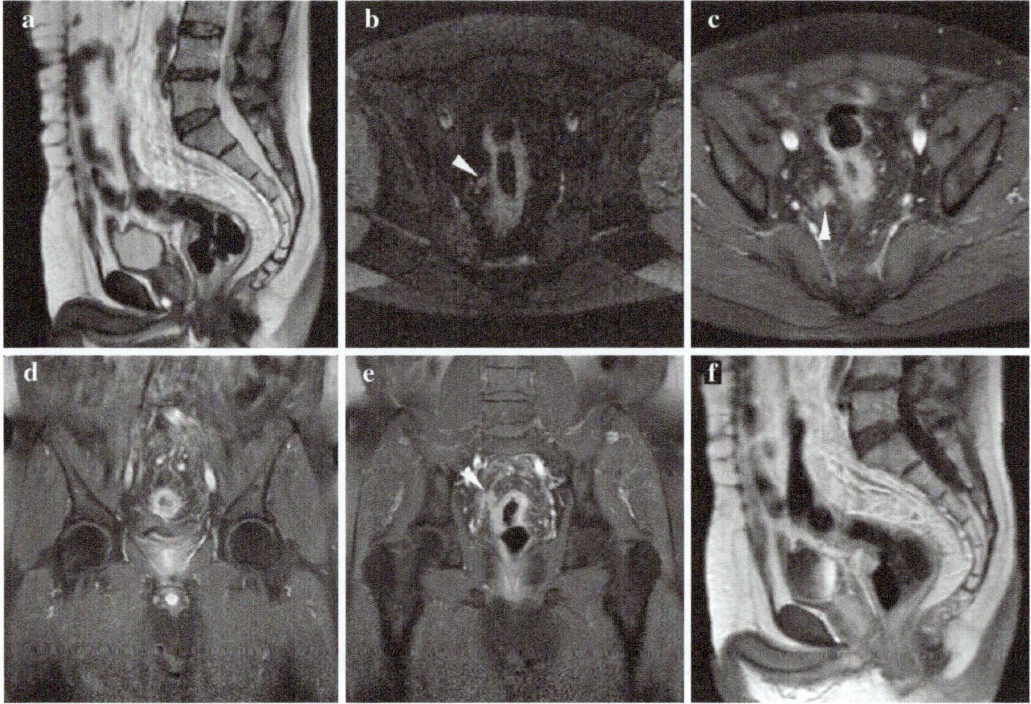

Fig. 10.2 60-year-old male patient with ulcerative colitis and endoscopic detection of rectosigmoid carcinoma. MRI including sagittal T2- (**a**), axial STIR (**b**) and post-contrast fat-suppressed (**c–e**) and unsuppressed (**f**) T1-weighted images effectively depicts 6-cm long circumferential full-thickness mural thickening, with strong contrast enhancement, irregular external margins, and at least one nodal metastasis (*arrowheads*) in the perivisceral fat

and the distance of the tumour from the key anatomic landmark represented by the mesorectal fascia [19, 20].

10.2 Low Rectal and Anal Carcinoma

An increased risk of anus and lower rectum carcinomas has been reported in patients with long-standing, severe perianal fistulizing Crohn's disease (CD) . In patients with CD, anal cancer occurs 20 years earlier than the general population, and reaches a 14 % proportion among all colorectal tumours, which is ten times

higher than the usual figure. However exceptionally, anal tumours may occasionally develop also in patients with ulcerative colitis (UC)-related chronic perianal inflammation (Fig. 10.3). The hypothesized pathogenesis involves an easier access of Human Papillomavirus to the anal epithelial layers due to fistulas, and chronic mucosal regeneration ultimately leading to neoplastic changes [21, 22].

The diagnosis of anal carcinoma in patients with IBD is usually unsuspected or delayed because of the pre-existent, unspecific complaints and because clinical assessment is hampered by complex inflammation with stricture and local pain. As a result, IBD-associated anal cancers are often advanced at presentation, may

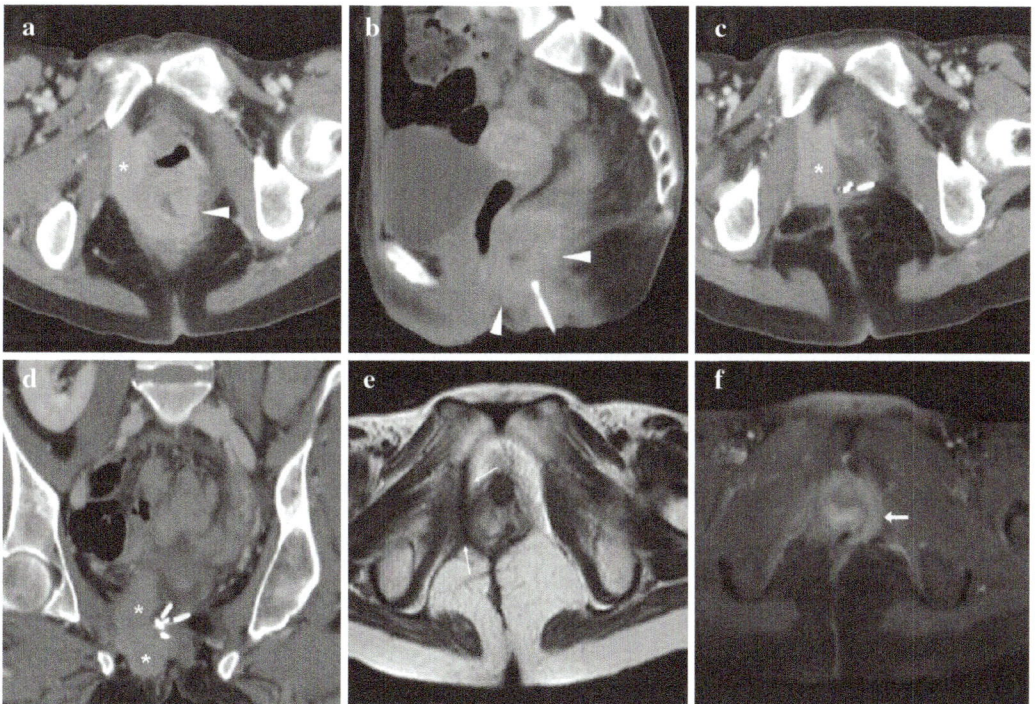

Fig. 10.3 39-year-old female with history of ulcerative colitis and perianal inflammation. Initial multiplanar MDCT (**a**, **b**) identified enhancing anal thickening (*arrowheads*) with *right*-sided vaginal infiltration and solid tissue (*) extending to reach the internal obturator muscle. After biopsy confirmation of SCAC and surgical debulking with colostomy, repeat MDCT (**c**, **d**) detected enlarging neoplastic residue (*). Shortly after chemoradiotherapy, MRI (**e**) detected the formation of a thick

hypointense fibrotic band in the site of the regressed tumour (*thin arrows*). MRI follow-up (**f**) identified appearance of a contralateral enhancing tissue band interpreted as suspicious for local recurrence (*arrow*). After negative clinical reassessment and PET findings, this post-treatment finding remained stable on further MRI studies (not shown) (reprinted from *Open Access* Ref. no. 24)

require extensive surgery plus chemo- and radiotherapy, and are associated with a severe prognosis [21–23].

Therefore, patients with long-standing IBD-related perianal inflammatory disease should undergo clinical and imaging surveillance, particularly when new or changed symptoms develop. Radiologists should be aware of the increased risk for anorectal cancer in middle-aged IBD patients, and clearly report any solid tissue as suspicious for neoplasm and suggest biopsy [21–24].

Currently, MRI represents the imaging modality of choice for primary regional staging of anal cancer. Solid neoplastic tissue shows low- to intermediate T1 signal intensity, T2- and STIR hypersignal superior to the internal reference standard represented by uninvolved anal sphincters and gluteal muscles, and positive enhancement after intravenous gadolinium contrast. Although with limited sensitivity compared to MRI, on CT images anal cancer may be detected as solid, enhancing nodules or masses within the anus, with progressive heterogeneity with increasing size [24–26].

As recommended by the European Society for Medical Oncology (ESMO), MRI is the primary imaging modality to accurately stage anal cancer taking into account the maximum tumour diameter, possible invasion of adjacent organs and nodal involvement. After radio-chemotherapy, imaging follow-up with MRI complements clinical evaluation in the assessment of therapeutic response, and of possible recurrences [24–26].

References

1. Zisman TL, Rubin DT (2008) Colorectal cancer and dysplasia in inflammatory bowel disease. World J Gastroenterol 14:2662–2669
2. Biancone L, Michetti P, Travis S et al (2008) European evidence-based consensus on the management of ulcerative colitis: special situations. J Crohns Colitis 2:63–92
3. Rutter MD, Saunders BP, Wilkinson KH et al (2006) Thirty-year analysis of a colonoscopic surveillance program for neoplasia in ulcerative colitis. Gastroenterology 130:1030–1038
4. Van Assche G, Dignass A, Bokemeyer B et al (2013) Second European evidence-based consensus on the diagnosis and management of ulcerative colitis part 3: special situations. J Crohns Colitis 7:1–33
5. Stange EF, Travis SP, Vermeire S et al (2008) European evidence-based Consensus on the diagnosis and management of ulcerative colitis: definitions and diagnosis. J Crohns Colitis 2:1–23
6. Dignass A, Eliakim R, Magro F et al (2012) Second European evidence-based consensus on the diagnosis and management of ulcerative colitis part 1: definitions and diagnosis. J Crohns Colitis 6:965–990
7. Mpofu C, Watson AJ, Rhodes JM (2004) Strategies for detecting colon cancer and/or dysplasia in patients with inflammatory bowel disease. Cochrane Database Syst Rev:CD000279
8. Efthymiou M, Taylor AC, Kamm MA (2011) Cancer surveillance strategies in ulcerative colitis: the need for modernization. Inflamm Bowel Dis 17: 1800–1813
9. Goetz M, Neurath MF (2009) Imaging techniques in inflammatory bowel disease: recent trends, questions and answers. Gastroenterol Clin Biol 33(Suppl 3): S174–S182
10. Ahmadi A, Polyak S, Draganov PV (2009) Colorectal cancer surveillance in inflammatory bowel disease: the search continues. World J Gastroenterol 15:61–66
11. Hristova L, Soyer P, Hoeffel C, et al (2012) Colorectal cancer in inflammatory bowel diseases: CT features with pathological correlation. Abdom Imaging 38:421–435
12. Levine MS, Rubesin SE, Laufer I et al (2000) Diagnosis of colorectal neoplasms at double-contrast barium enema examination. Radiology 216:11–18
13. Ridereau-Zins C, Aube C, Luet D et al (2010) Assessment of water enema computed tomography: an effective imaging technique for the diagnosis of colon cancer: colon cancer: computed tomography using a water enema. Abdom Imaging 35:407–413
14. Soyer P, Sirol M, Dray X, et al (2012) Detection of colorectal tumors with water enema-multidetector row computed tomography. Abdom Imaging 37:1092–1100
15. Ridereau-Zins C, Sibileau E, Pavageau AH, et al (2011) Accuracy of water enema-MDCT in colon cancer staging: a prospective study. Cancer Imaging 11(Spec No A):S115
16. Regge D, Neri E, Turini F et al (2009) Role of CT colonography in inflammatory bowel disease. Eur J Radiol 69:404–408
17. Soyer P, Hamzi L, Sirol M et al (2012) Colon cancer: comprehensive evaluation with 64-section CT colonography using water enema as intraluminal contrast agent-a pictorial review. Clin Imaging 36:113–125
18. Stabile Ianora AA, Moschetta M, Pedote P et al (2012) Preoperative local staging of colosigmoideal cancer: air versus water multidetector-row CT colonography. Radiol Med 117:254–267

19. Klessen C, Rogalla P, Taupitz M (2007) Local staging of rectal cancer: the current role of MRI. Eur Radiol 17:379–389
20. Torkzad MR, Pahlman L, Glimelius B (2010) Magnetic resonance imaging (MRI) in rectal cancer: a comprehensive review. Insights Imaging 1:245–267
21. Ky A, Sohn N, Weinstein MA et al (1998) Carcinoma arising in anorectal fistulas of Crohn's disease. Dis Colon Rectum 41:992–996
22. Sjodahl RI, Myrelid P, Soderholm JD (2003) Anal and rectal cancer in Crohn's disease. Colorectal Dis 5:490–495
23. Devon KM, Brown CJ, Burnstein M et al (2009) Cancer of the anus complicating perianal Crohn's disease. Dis Colon Rectum 52:211–216
24. Tonolini M, Bianco R (2013) MRI and CT of anal carcinoma: a pictorial review. Insights Imaging
25. Roach SC, Hulse PA, Moulding FJ et al (2005) Magnetic resonance imaging of anal cancer. Clin Radiol 60:1111–1119
26. Kochhar R, Plumb AA, Carrington BM et al (2012) Imaging of anal carcinoma. Am J Roentgenol 199:W335–W344

Musculoskeletal Manifestations of Ulcerative Colitis

11

Roberto Bianco and Massimo Tonolini

11.1 Introduction

Affecting approximately 35–40 % of patients, musculoskeletal complications associated with Ulcerative Colitis (UC) are considered the most frequent extraintestinal manifestations of inflammatory bowel diseases (IBD), and include inflammatory conditions characteristically involving the axial skeleton, the peripheral joints or a combination of these, along with other extra-articular conditions [1–3].

By far the commonest musculoskeletal manifestation, UC-related arthropathies, affect both sexes but are more frequently encountered in males, and can be categorized according to the involvement of the axial skeleton or peripheral joints [2–4].

Axial IBD-associated (or enteropathic) arthropathy includes sacroiliitis and spondyloarthritis (SpA), and is classified as one of the five subtypes of serum-negative spondyloarthropathies, a group of distinct disorders sharing similar clinical features and a common genetic predisposition, along with ankylosing spondylitis (AS), psoriatic arthritis, reactive (Reiter's) arthritis and undifferentiated SpA [2].

Enteropathic SpA is diagnosed clinically with fair sensitivity and specificity on the basis of the presence of inflammatory back pain (IBP), that characteristically occurs in patients under 40 years of age, is frequently insidious in onset, worsens at night and is relieved by exercise but does not improve with rest [2]. According to the revised Rome criteria, the diagnosis of AS includes chronic IBP, morning stiffness, limited spinal flexion and reduced chest expansion in its most advanced stages [5]. In patients with UC, AS has a prevalence of 4–10 %. Positivity for the HLA-B27 histocompatibility antigen is correlated with susceptibility for developing SpA, and is found in 25–75 % of patients with UC and AS, but in only 7–15 % of patients with UC and isolated sacroiliitis [3, 6–8].

Sacroiliitis can be diagnosed on the basis of associated classic radiographic criteria established since 1966, and presence of inflammatory low back pain, including at least four of the five Calin's criteria (presentation before 40 years, insidious onset, improvement with exercise, morning stiffness and persistence of symptoms for at least 3 months) [9]. Although sacroiliitis is reported to affect 10–20 % of UC patients, asymptomatic radiographic changes suggesting sacroiliitis are increasingly recognized in up to 25–50 % of them, particularly because of the improved sensitivity intrinsic to Magnetic Resonance Imaging (MRI) [1, 3, 6, 10].

R. Bianco (✉)
Head, Radiology Department, "Luigi Sacco" University Hospital, Via G.B. Grassi 74, 20157 Milan, Italy
e-mail: bianco.roberto@hsacco.it

M. Tonolini
Radiology Department, "Luigi Sacco" University Hospital, Via G.B. Grassi 74, 20157 Milan, Italy
e-mail: mtonolini@sirm.org

M. Tonolini (ed.), *Imaging of Ulcerative Colitis*,
DOI: 10.1007/978-88-470-5409-7_11, © Springer-Verlag Italia 2014

Peripheral arthritis, either in the form of oligo- or poliarticular involvement, is less frequent than axial arthropathy and occurs in 8–29 % of patients. The Oxford classification categorizes peripheral arthropathy into type I and type II, with only the former associated with intestinal disease activity. Affecting 4–17 % of patients with UC, type I is an oligoarthritis which affects asymmetrically the large, weight-bearing joints such as the knees, ankles, hips, wrists and sometimes the elbows and shoulders, with the knee being the most frequently affected site. Clinically, it is characterized by acute although self-limited flares with joint tenderness, swelling and functional impairment. The more uncommon type II affects 2.5 % of UC patients, is a polyarticular arthritis independent of IBD activity that affects more than five joints, particularly the metacarpophalangeal and interphalangeal joints of the hands and feet, occasionally the knees, ankles and shoulders [3, 6, 11].

Other musculoskeletal manifestations include enthesitis, corresponding to inflammatory processes of the tendons, ligaments and joint capsule insertions at the bone, which most usually affects the Achilles tendon, followed by the plantar fascia and patellar tendon; dactylitis, characterized by inflammatory swelling of one or more fingers due to tenosynovitis of the flexor tendons; and chest pain from enthesitis of the costovertebral, costosternal, manubrio-costal joints exacerbated by coughing and deep breaths [2].

Furthermore, low mineral bone from metabolic disturbances is common (20–50 %) in both male and female patients suffering from UC. Contributing factors include chronic systemic inflammation, corticosteroid therapy, ageing, cigarette smoking, limited physical activity, nutritional vitamin D deficiency, low dietary calcium intake, decreased serum levels of albumin and ileal resorption [3, 6, 12].

The overall fracture risk in patients with UC has been estimated at 1 per 100 patient-years, which is 40 % higher than that of the general population, and the risk increases with age. Osteopenia and osteoporosis are diagnosed by means of Dual Energy X-ray Absorptiometry (DEXA) bone densitometry, on the basis of a T

score below −1 or below −2.5, respectively, and can identify patients with increased or markedly increased risk for fracture. DEXA scanning is advised in patients with persistently active UC, history of steroid therapy and/or long-standing disease [3, 6, 12].

11.2 Imaging Axial Arthropathy with MRI

In patients affected with UC, the association of conventional radiographs and MRI allows comprehensive visualization (or otherwise exclusion) and staging of inflammatory changes in the axial skeleton [13, 14].

Currently, MRI is considered the gold standard imaging modality to detect inflammatory changes in the spine and in the sacroiliac joints. Whereas radiographic changes usually develop 5 years after the onset of symptoms, MRI is the most sensitive diagnostic technique in early, active phases because of its ability to demonstrate inflammation before radiographically identifiable bone lesions develop. MRI has a sensitivity and specificity of 90 %, which becomes even higher with correct acquisition protocol and interpretation by radiologists familiar with rheumatologic disorders [3, 4, 6, 15]. Furthermore, being reproducible MRI allows confident reassessment of inflammatory changes following disease-modifying pharmacological treatment, since reduction in oedematous spinal changes is consistent with therapeutic response [14].

11.2.1 Spine

Imaging the spine in patients with clinically suspected or confirmed enteropathic SpA involves panoramic acquisition of the entire cervical, dorsal and lumbosacral segments, which should be nowadays performed on high-magnetic field (1–1.5 Tesla) MRI scanners. Because of the subtlety of most MRI findings, detection and characterization of acute and chronic inflammatory abnormalities rely on a correct acquisition protocol. Unenhanced

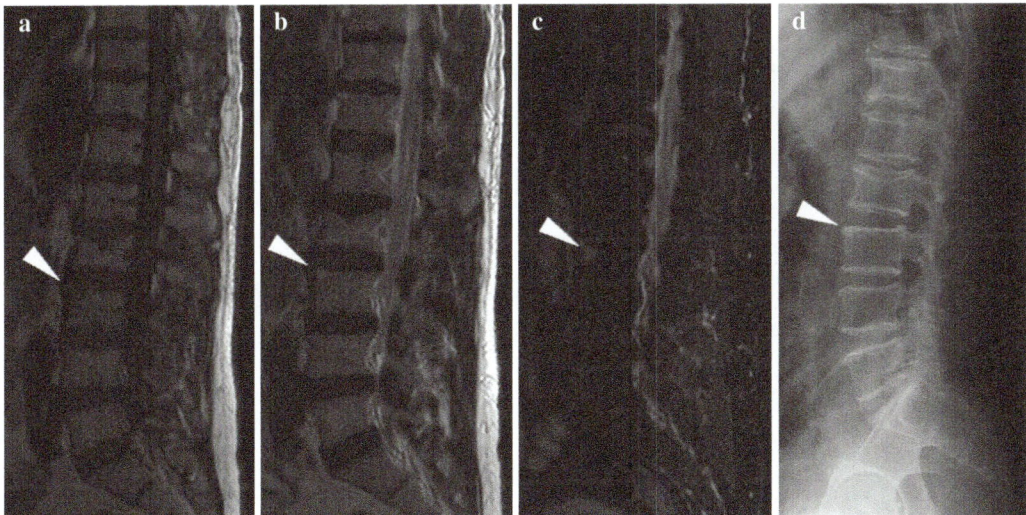

Fig. 11.1 Acute spondylitis. Unenhanced sagittal T1- (**a**), T2-weighted (**b**) and STIR (**c**) MRI images show triangular abnormality at the *upper* anterior corner of the L2 vertebral body (*arrowheads*), with low T1-, high T2- and STIR signal intensity consistent with the presence of bone marrow oedema (focal osteitis). In the same patient, a latero-lateral radiograph (**d**) shows corresponding sclerotic marginal irregularity (*arrowhead*)

sagittal-oriented T1-, T2-weighted Turbo Spin Echo (TSE) and fat-suppressed T2 or STIR (short tau inversion recovery) sequences should be acquired, followed by additional transverse (axial) images focused on abnormal findings. Optional T1-weighted acquisition with fat saturation after intravenous administration of paramagnetic gadolinium-based contrast medium is recommended in selected cases, particularly to distinguish aseptic inflammation from infectious spondylodiskitis [4, 14].

Inflammatory changes in the bony spine include spondylitis, spondylodiskitis, arthritis of the facet joints, costovertebral arthritis and enthesitis of the spinal ligaments. The vertebral involvement may follow or precede the appearance of the sacroiliitis; however, most usually both lesions are detected simultaneously [4, 8].

The key abnormality consistent with spinal involvement is represented by spondylitis. In their earliest, active phases the classical lesions, initially described by Romanus, are not radiographically appreciable. Conversely, at MRI they show up as small, triangular T1-hypointense, T2- and STIR-hyperintense signal abnormalities with perceptible enhancement on post-contrast fat-saturated T1-weighted sequences, located at one or more anterior or posterior vertebral corners in the insertion site of the annulus fibrosus, representing bone marrow oedema (BME) or focal "osteitis" (Figs. 11.1, 11.2a). These changes are observed in 67 % of patients with SpA. The specificity for SpA is 81 % when more than three corners are involved, and reaches 97 % if the patient is below 40 years of age [4, 8, 16].

Alternatively, the inflammatory (non-infectious) spondylodiskitis or Andersson lesion is observed in 33 % of patients with SpA, and characterized by hemispherically shaped BME signal abnormalities along two facing vertebral endplates [4]. Although less common, other possible imaging appearances of enteropathic SpA include arthritis of the synovial joints of the column, characterized by the presence of BME in the facet, costovertebral or costotransverse joints, and enthesitis of the spinal ligaments heralded by high STIR signal intensity and contrast enhancement at the insertion sites of the supraspinous and interspinous ligaments [14].

In later stages of the spinal inflammatory process, BME changes along somatic edges undergo adipose degeneration, leading to a hyperintense appearance on both T1- and

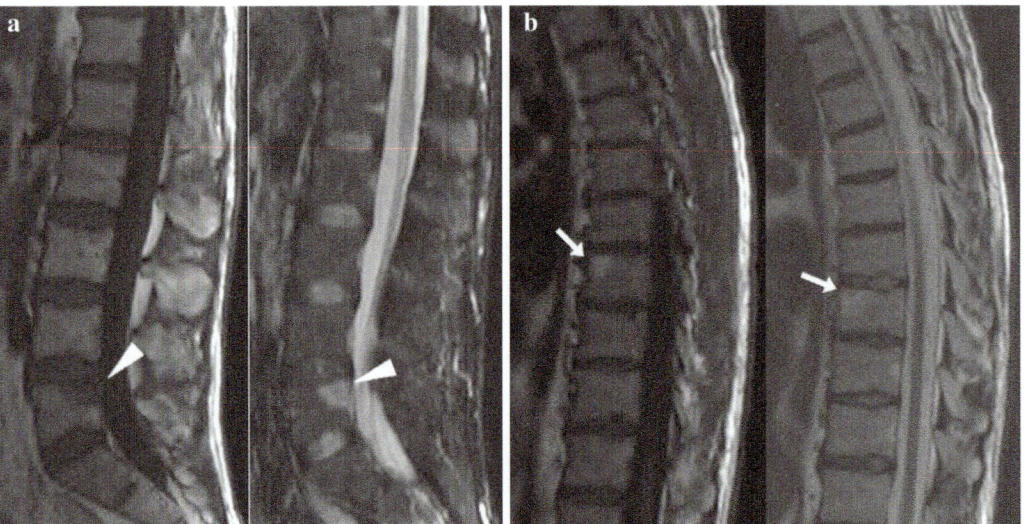

Fig. 11.2 Mixed acute and chronic spondylitis changes. Unenhanced sagittal T1- (**a**) and STIR (**b**) MRI images of the lumbar spine, respectively, show hypo- and hyperintense signal abnormalities (*arrowheads*) at the upper posterior corner of the L5 vertebral body, indicating the presence of bone marrow edema and consistent with active spondylitis. In the same patient, T1- (**c**) and T2-weighted (**d**) MRI images of the dorsal tract show hyperintense signal in both sequences (*arrows*) at an upper anterior vertebral body corner, indicating adipose bone marrow replacement and consistent with chronic spondylitis

T2-weighted sequences with corresponding hypointensity with fat suppression techniques. This post-inflammatory fatty bone marrow replacement is consistent with chronic spondylitis (Fig. 11.2b). Furthermore, these deposits are strongly predictive of the formation of syndesmophytes. In fact, this phase coincides with the initial radiographic appearance of syndesmophytes, which represent newly formed thin, vertically oriented bony structures at the level of the vertebral bodies corners at the edge of the disks. Finally, in more advanced phases sclerosis, new bone formation and ankylosis may develop. The appearance of bone marrow adipose deposition and of bony bridges across the intervertebral disk represents spinal ankylosis in long-standing disease [4, 13, 14].

11.2.2 Sacroiliac Joints

Predominantly composed of fibrous connective tissue with very little synovial fluid, the sacroiliac joints are considered enthesis, and as such are characteristically involved in axial SpA [15].

Although plain radiographs are usually obtained as the initial imaging test, their role is limited to the assessment of mineral and cortical bone changes. On the other hand, MRI allows visualizing the cartilage and bone marrow changes. Similarly to the spine, MRI is superior for the assessment of active inflammatory changes, making it possible to diagnose sacroiliitis earlier, before definite joint degeneration becomes radiographically visible. As such, MRI of the sacroiliac joints is necessary to confirm acute involvement, and to assess post-treatment modifications [13, 15].

A typical MRI acquisition protocol should include T1-weighted and STIR images along the proper oblique-coronal plane and oblique-axial T1- and T2-weighted images, oriented, respectively, parallel and perpendicular to the main longitudinal axis of the sacroiliac joints.

Either uni- or bilateral, inflammatory changes of the sacroiliac joints are detected by MRI with imaging findings that closely resemble those described in the spine. Early, active sacroiliitis is heralded by the MRI identification of BME on the subchondral bone, which appears as a

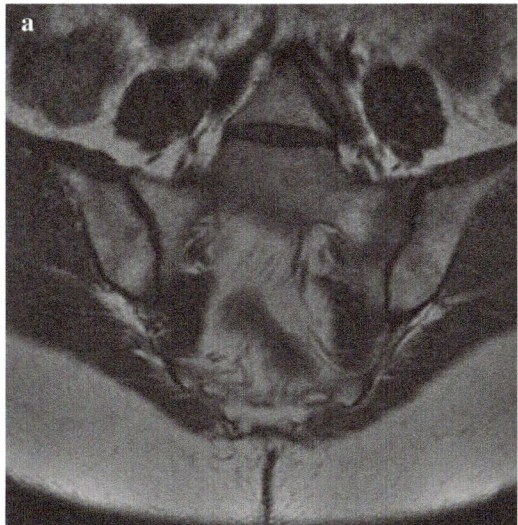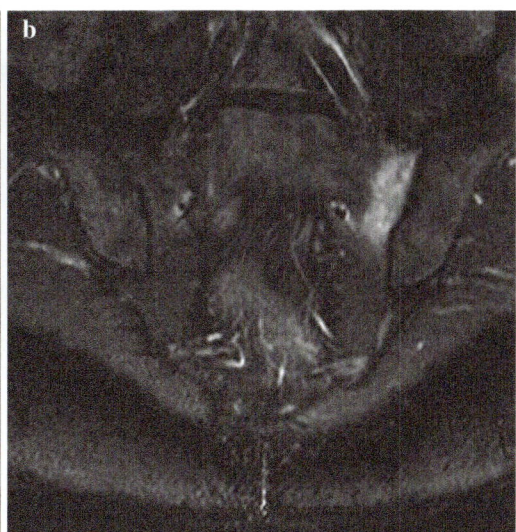

Fig. 11.3 Acute sacroiliitis. Unenhanced oblique coronal T1-weighted (**a**) and STIR (**b**) MRI images show extensive hypo- and hyperintense signal subchondral band abnormality along the sacral aspect of the left sacroiliac joint, indicating the presence of bone marrow edema from active inflammation

circumscribed periarticular area of low T1-, high T2- and STIR signal intensity (Fig. 11.3). Initially, BME can be found on the iliac or sacral side only, but typically becomes bilateral and symmetric on both sides of the involved joint, and characteristically located at its lower and posterior thirds. When unilateral, differentiation from infectious sacroiliitis may be challenging. Stronger STIR hypersignal more likely reflects pronounced disease activity, and active subchondral bone changes are seen to enhance when fat-saturated T1-weighted images are acquired after intravenous contrast [4, 16].

Later in the course of the disease, inflammation subsides and progressive post-inflammatory fatty marrow degeneration occurs, which appears hyperintense on both T1- and T2-weighted sequences with signal drop on fat-suppressed images (Fig. 11.4a, b). Furthermore, chronic sacroiliitis includes subchondral sclerosis on both iliac and sacral surfaces that is depicted with low signal intensity and without enhancement, and typically extends at least 5 mm from the articular surface. Isolated or confluent erosions may be identifiable, represented by bony defects with low signal intensity on T1-weighted images on the articular surface. Finally, joint space narrowing develops, ultimately leading to articular fusion. Whereas cortical bone changes and the joint space are better depicted by computed tomography (CT), ankylosis of the sacroiliac joints is exquisitely diagnosed at MRI when bridging bone marrow is seen between the fused iliac wing and sacrum (Fig. 11.4c, d) [4].

11.3 Imaging Axial Arthropathy with Conventional Radiology

As discussed earlier in this chapter, plain radiographs have limited diagnostic value in the early stages of axial SpA.

11.3.1 Spine

The classic Romanus lesion represents the hallmark of radiographic vertebral involvement, and includes focal irregularity, erosion and/or sclerosis at the anterior and/or posterior edges of the vertebral endplate, corresponding to the site of attachment of the annulus fibrosus and of insertion of the vertebral ligaments (Fig. 11.1d). Subsequently, new bone formation leads to the

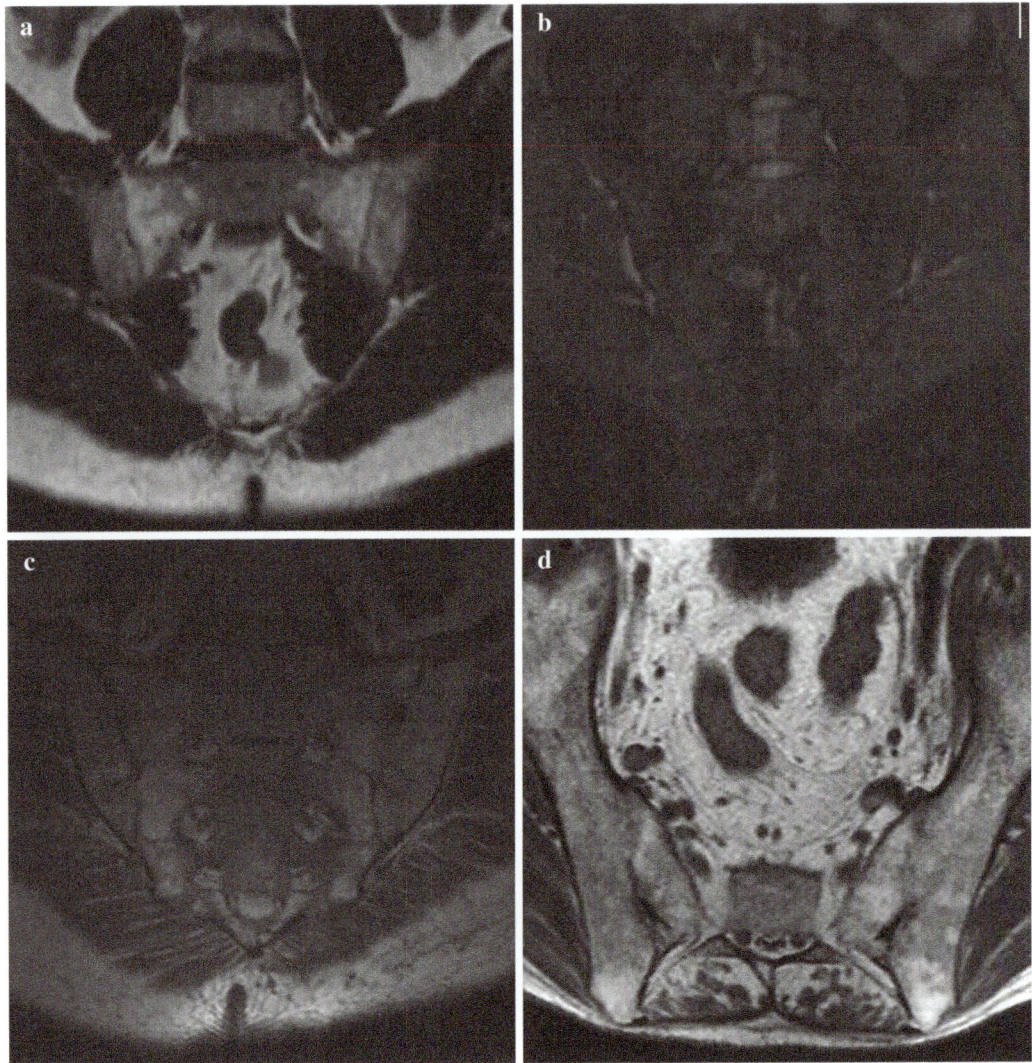

Fig. 11.4 Chronic sacroiliitis. Unenhanced oblique coronal T1-weighted (**a**) and STIR (**b**) MRI images show extensive T1-hyperintense bone marrow signal changes in both sacral wings, with corresponding low signal intensity with fat suppression, consistent with adipose marrow replacement. The sacroiliac joint spaces are narrowed. In a different patient, oblique-coronal (**c**) and axial (**d**) T1-weighted images show similar extensive adipose bone marrow changes along both lateral aspects of the sacrum, whereas the joint space is occupied by bridging bone marrow indicating ankylosis

appearance of thin, vertically oriented syndesmophytes at the periphery of disks, most usually symmetric and bilateral (Fig. 11.5). In long-standing SpA, widespread syndesmophytosis results in the characteristic "bamboo spine" appearance [4, 8, 16].

Chronic inflammatory bony changes to the spine are even better depicted by CT, and the same is true for syndesmophytes (Fig. 11.5), which despite a characteristic appearance on plain radiographs, are unreliably identified by MRI [13, 14].

11.3.2 Sacroiliac Joints

A focused radiological study of the sacroiliac joints should include antero-posterior projection

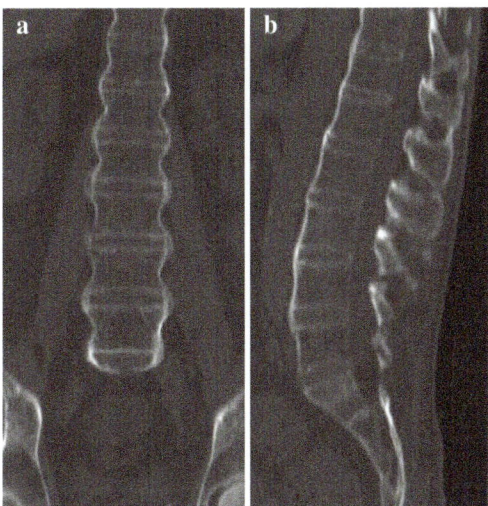

Fig. 11.5 Extensive syndesmophytosis of the spine. Unenhanced coronal (**a**) and sagittal (**b**) multiplanar CT reformations show diffuse lumbar spine involvement by thin, vertically oriented syndesmophytes along both sides of the intervertebral disk spaces with preserved height

views with an incident beam angled 20–30° in cranio-caudal direction. The classical radiographic signs of sacroiliitis include pseudo-extension of the joint space, iuxta-articular osteoporosis, followed by erosive changes and subchondral osteosclerosis in later stages.

The radiological staging of sacroiliitis is based on the New York criteria that include five categories: Grade 0 is normal appearance, Grade 1 corresponds to slightly blurred joint edges, narrowing, or pseudo-extension of the joint space and mild subchondral sclerosis. Grade 2 includes irregularities of the articular margins with evidence of erosion, joint space narrowing and evident subchondral sclerosis, whereas Grade 3 involves articular erosions and evident subchondral sclerosis with initial synostotic bridges. Finally, Grade 4 corresponds to complete sacroiliac ankylosis.

Because of the uncertainties intrinsic to plain radiograph interpretation, related to the anatomical complexity of the sacroiliac joints, CT is helpful to clarify early bony changes such as erosions and sclerosis, with the possibility of generating focused oblique-axial and coronal image reformations. Conversely, in advanced

sacroiliitis with ankylosis CT has similar sensitivity to conventional radiology.

11.4   Differential Diagnosis of Axial Arthropathy

Concerning the spine, the differential diagnosis of SpA include osteophytes in dorso-lumbar osteoarthritis, which should not be confused with syndesmophytes because they are thicker bone proliferations that grow horizontally from the endplate and subsequently coalesce to form a coarse bony bridge between the vertebral endplates. Conversely, syndesmophytes are thinner and have a vertical orientation, extending bilaterally and symmetrically between two vertebral bodies. Furthermore, an exuberant "flowing" prevertebral ossification along multiple vertebral bodies is observed in diffuse idiopathic skeletal hyperostosis (DISH). The degenerative Modic I (representing inflammation) and Modic II (representing conversion to yellow adipose marrow) changes may not always be easily differentiated from Andersson lesions, although they are usually associated with degenerative process of the intervertebral disk. Finally, infectious spondylodiskitis may have a similar appearance, including high signal intensity on fat-suppressed and STIR images along the vertebral endplates; however, clinical and laboratory hints to the diagnosis are usually present, the vertebral body contour is disrupted and the involved disk shows prominent signal and enhancement changes. The surrounding soft tissue and/or epidural space are often involved with or without abscess collections [4, 17, 18].

Differential diagnoses of enteropathic sacroiliitis include degenerative changes in the sacroiliac joints, characterized by irregularity and narrowing of the articular space, juxta-articular sclerosis, that are usually found in the anterior and middle thirds and do not include inflammatory changes such as erosions. Associated with fever and characteristic laboratory abnormalities, infectious sacroiliitis is unilateral in most cases, with signal and enhancement changes in the articular surfaces, associated surrounding soft tissue involvement and sometimes abscess formation. Finally, osteitis condensans ilii, a benign radiographic appearance most usually found in multiparous women, involves triangular areas of sclerosis unilateral or bilateral to the iliac bone [4, 19, 20].

11.5 Imaging Peripheral Arthropathy

In most cases, the diagnosis of UC-associated non-axial arthropathy is made on clinical grounds, based on the characteristic finding of painful swollen joints and exclusion of other specific forms of arthritis such as osteoarthritis, rheumatoid arthritis and arthritis associated with connective tissue diseases. Furthermore, complications of treatment for UC such as corticosteroid-related osteonecrosis should be excluded [3, 6].

As noted above, in type I peripheral arthropathy the knee is the most frequently affected joint. Ultrasound initially shows distension of the joint capsule and effusion, and in later stages thickening of the synovial membrane. Power-Doppler sonography may be helpful to distinguish the solid, vascularized proliferative component from fluid, which is devoid of vascular signals [8]. On plain radiographs, the affected joint shows a symmetrical reduction of the articular space, juxta-articular osteoporosis, and small and late bone erosions. At MRI, fluid distension of the joint capsule and BME changes in the articular surfaces are detected, best on fat-suppressed T2-weighted or STIR images, with corresponding enhancement after intravenous contrast medium administration. In rare instances, progression to ankylosis may occur at the level of the peripheral joints too [8].

11.6 Imaging Entheses

As mentioned above, the most common enthesitis include Achilles tendonitis, plantar fasciitis and patellar tendon inflammation. The diagnosis is clinical, and can be confirmed by means of B-mode and power-Doppler sonography, or with MRI. Ultrasound can detect tendon thickening, tendinosis and peritendinitis, associated calcifications, bursitis and periosteal changes. Power Doppler ultrasound allows to detect abnormal vascularization corresponding to acute inflammation of the tendons, bursae and tendon insertions at the bone cortex. At MRI, the hallmark of enthesitis is represented by the detection of BME at the interface between bone and tendons, along with inflammatory oedema of the surrounding soft tissues. Bursitis, increased signal of tendons and BME changes are best appreciated on T2-weighted sequences with fat suppression, and enhanced on post-contrast fat-saturated T1-weighted images. In their full-blown stages, conventional radiographs may show swelling of the enthesis, coarsely calcified enthesophytes, erosions and osteoporosis, bone sclerosis and deformity in tendon insertional sites [8].

References

1. Levine JS, Burakoff R (2011) Extraintestinal manifestations of inflammatory bowel disease. Gastroenterol Hepatol (N Y) 7:235–241
2. Salvarani C, Fries W (2009) Clinical features and epidemiology of spondyloarthritides associated with inflammatory bowel disease. World J Gastroenterol 15:2449–2455
3. Van Assche G, Dignass A, Bokemeyer B et al (2013) Second European evidence-based consensus on the diagnosis and management of ulcerative colitis Part III: special situations. J Crohns Colitis 7:1–33
4. Canella C, Schau B, Ribeiro E et al (2013) MRI in seronegative spondyloarthritis: imaging features and differential diagnosis in the spine and sacroiliac joints. AJR Am J Roentgenol 200:149–157
5. Kellgren JH, Jeffrey MR, Ball J (1963) The epidemiology of chronic rheumatism. Blackwell, Oxford, 623–627
6. Biancone L, Michetti P, Travis S et al (2008) European evidence-based consensus on the management of ulcerative colitis: special situations. J Crohns Colitis 2:63–92
7. de Vlam K, Mielants H, Cuvelier C et al (2000) Spondyloarthropathy is underestimated in inflammatory bowel disease: prevalence and HLA association. J Rheumatol 27:2860–2865

8. Garlaschi G, Martino F (2007) Artrite reumatoide e spondiloentesoartriti: diagnostica per immagini e imaging follow-up. Springer Verlag Italia

9. Calin A, Porta J, Fries JF et al (1977) Clinical history as a screening test for ankylosing spondylitis. JAMA 237:2613–2614

10. Queiro R, Maiz O, Intxausti J et al (2000) Subclinical sacroiliitis in inflammatory bowel disease: a clinical and follow-up study. Clin Rheumatol 19:445–449

11. Orchard TR, Wordsworth BP, Jewell DP (1998) Peripheral arthropathies in inflammatory bowel disease: their articular distribution and natural history. Gut 42:387–391

12. AGA (2003) American gastroenterological association medical position statement: guidelines on osteoporosis in gastrointestinal diseases. Gastroenterology 124:791–794

13. Lacout A, Rousselin B, Pelage JP (2008) CT and MRI of spine and sacroiliac involvement in spondyloarthropathy. AJR Am J Roentgenol 191: 1016–1023

14. Hermann KG, Althoff CE, Schneider U et al (2005) Spinal changes in patients with spondyloarthritis: comparison of MR imaging and radiographic appearances. Radiographics 25:559–569; discussion 569–570

15. Guglielmi G, Cascavilla A, Scalzo G et al (2011) Imaging findings of sacroiliac joints in spondyloarthropathies and other rheumatic conditions. Radiol Med 116:292–301

16. Sieper J, Rudwaleit M, Baraliakos X et al (2009) The assessment of spondylogrthritis international society (ASAS) handbook: a guide to assess spondyloarthritis. Ann Rheum Dis 68:ii1-ii44, (Suppl 2)

17. Longo M, Granata F, Ricciardi K et al (2003) Contrast-enhanced MR imaging with fat suppression in adult-onset septic spondylodiscitis. Eur Radiol 13:626–637

18. Rahme R, Moussa R (2008) The modic vertebral endplate and marrow changes: pathologic significance and relation to low back pain and segmental instability of the lumbar spine. AJNR Am J Neuroradiol 29:838–842

19. Jacobson JA, Girish G, Jiang Y et al (2008) Radiographic evaluation of arthritis: inflammatory conditions. Radiology 248:378–389

20. Jacobson JA, Girish G, Jiang Y et al (2008) Radiographic evaluation of arthritis: degenerative joint disease and variations. Radiology 248:737–747

Surgical Perspective on Perianal Complications in Ulcerative Colitis

12

Gianluca Matteo Sampietro, Francesco Colombo, Alice Frontali and Diego Foschi

12.1 Introduction

Perianal disease (PD) in Inflammatory Bowel Diseases (IBD) is typically associated with Crohn's disease (CD). In fact, the presence of PD, even in an established diagnosis of Ulcerative Colitis (UC), always rises in the clinician's mind the suspect of CD. However, historical series of UC patients from the 1950s and the 1960s reported an incidence of PD in the range of 20–25 %. These rates, of course, were misleading, since colonic CD and Indeterminate Colitis (IC) were first recognized in the 1960s and 1970s, respectively. Certainly, many patients supposed in the past to have UC and PD really had CD or IC, but to date, little is known about the real incidence of PD among UC patients that is considered to be of about 5–15 % [1–13].

G. M. Sampietro (✉)
Head of IBD Surgical Unit—Department of Surgery, "Luigi Sacco" University Hospital, Via GB Grassi, 74, 20157 Milan, Italy
e-mail: gianluca.sampietro@unimi.it

F. Colombo · A. Frontali
Division of General Surgery—Department of Surgery, "Luigi Sacco" University Hospital, Via GB Grassi, 74, 20157 Milan, Italy
e-mail: colombo.francesco@hsacco.it

A. Frontali
e-mail: frontali.alice@hsacco.it

D. Foschi
Head of the Department of Surgery, "Luigi Sacco" University Hospital, Via GB Grassi, 74, 20157 Milan, Italy
e-mail: diego.foschi@unimi.it

12.2 Diagnosis and Management

Diagnosis of perianal complications in UC patients is crucial for deciding the most adequate therapeutic strategy. Since different diagnostic and therapeutic options are available in the treatment of PD, a global strategy should always be followed: control of sepsis, through abscess drainage and loose seton placement; sphincter preservation, by limiting damage to anal and perineal tissues; evaluation of the inflammation, due to its implication in further treatment; immunosuppression, on the basis of clinical needing.

The presence of a perianal abscess should be ruled out by clinical examination before any further investigation, and if present it should be drained as a matter of urgency (see later) (Fig. 12.1).

The two main aspects to be considered at the very beginning for their therapeutic and prognostic implications are the anatomical definition of the fistulous track(s) with associated complications, and the level of inflammation of the colon and rectum. For initial diagnosis of perianal fistulising UC, contrast-enhanced MRI should be considered the procedure of choice; Endoscopic Ultrasound (EUS) has similar sensitivity, but inferior specificity than MRI, and it cannot be performed in the presence of stenosis

M. Tonolini (ed.), *Imaging of Ulcerative Colitis*,
DOI: 10.1007/978-88-470-5409-7_12, © Springer-Verlag Italia 2014

Fig. 12.1 Drainage of a wide abscess of the whole right perineal region and silicone loose seton positioning in two fistula tracks

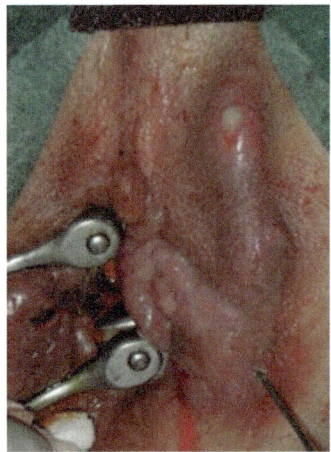
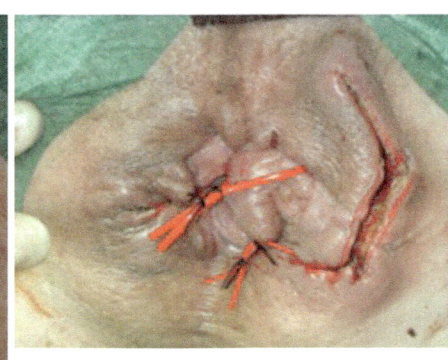

Fig. 12.1 Drainage of a wide abscess of the whole right perineal region and silicone loose seton positioning in two fistula tracks

and painful abscesses; Transperineal Ultrasound (TPUS) should be used in the presence of anal stenosis or abscesses, and both US methods can be improved with hydrogen peroxide enhancement; Computed Tomography (CT) is preferred in emergency settings. Fistulography is no more recommended. All these methods achieve the best results when combined with Examination Under Anaesthetics (EUA). EUA is reported to have an accuracy of 90 % in the hands of an experienced colorectal surgeon, but most important, it permits contemporary identification of all fistulae tracts, loose seton positioning and abscess drainage (Figs. 12.1 and 12.2) [14].

In CD patients, the incidence of perineal disease is 20–25 % in association with terminal ileitis, and it rises as high as 60 % for colonic location and 92 % when the rectum is actively involved. However, in UC patients the rectum is involved by definition, and thus a colonoscopy has to be performed in order to characterize the activity and the extension of the disease [14, 15].

Once a diagnosis of PD is established, there is no consensus for classifying the fistulae. The Parks' classification should be used for the description of fistulae courses due to its implication in surgical management, but in clinical practice most experts prefer the classification into simple or complex [14, 16]. Simple perianal fistula should be considered a fistula with a straight course connecting the internal and external orifices. Complex perianal fistulae are those with one or more of the following characteristics: multiple internal and/or external orifices; presence of ramifications with external orifices, with genitalia or blind sinuses in the perineal tissues; concomitant abscess, both as a mass or a circular collection between the muscles (horseshoe abscess); upper rectum, presacral, obturatory abscesses or phlegmons;

Fig. 12.2 EUA and loose seton positioning for stabilization of a perianal fistula. *Left*, identification of the track using a probe. *Right*, silicone loose seton in position

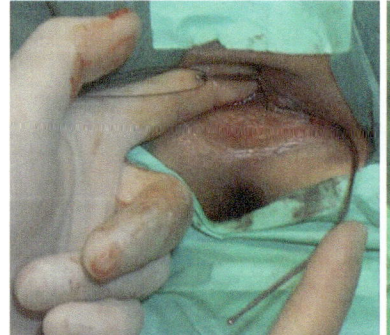
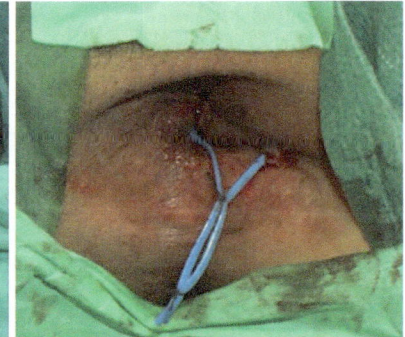

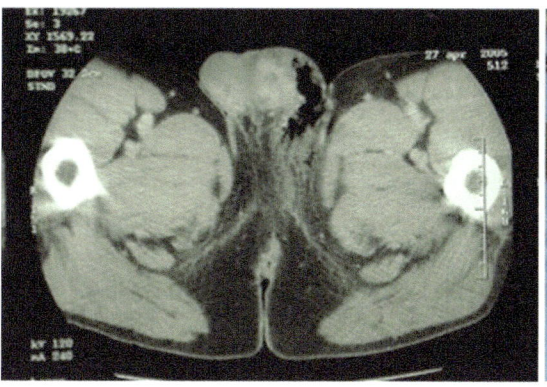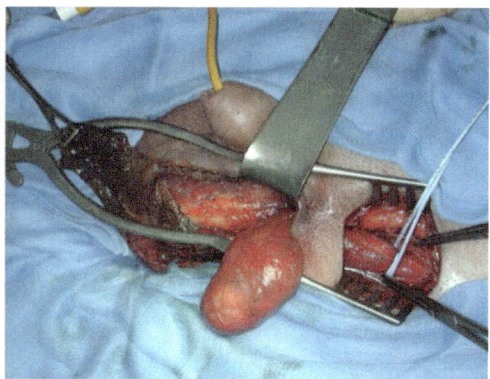

Fig. 12.3 55-year-old male UC patient presenting with Fournier's gangrene. The patient was under high-dose steroids treatment due to a recent episode of acute colitis. *Left*, urgent CT scan at admission. *Right*, emergency surgical procedure with complete exposure of the inguinal and scrotal regions. The left testis was isolated and preserved, while the left scrotum was completely destroyed

single or concomitant ano-vaginal and recto-vaginal tracts; concomitant severe rectal inflammation. Furthermore, a pelvic floor dysfunction should be addressed and, in case of severe pelvic muscles impairment, a specific rehabilitation programme should be adopted (pelvic floor dysfunction is responsible for several perianal problems in the general population, so it should be excluded as an additional risk factor for PD diagnosis and treatment).

Simple perianal fistulae should be treated only if symptomatic. In case of treatment, loose seton placement and/or antibiotics (metronidazole and ciprofloxacin) should be indicated.

Complex fistulae should always be treated with abscess drainage and loose seton placement. The time of seton removal depends on subsequent medical therapy. In case of active luminal disease, a concomitant pharmacological treatment is indicated. Antibiotics (metronidazole and ciprofloxacin) in association with immunomodulators (azathioprine, 6-mercaptopurine, tacrolimus, etc.) or biological (infliximab or adalimumab) are the treatment of choice. Uncontrolled perianal sepsis in UC patients under steroids and/or immunosuppressant treatment could lead to Fournier's gangrene, a rapidly progressive, life-threatening condition that requires emergency surgery (Fig. 12.3) [17].

In case a total proctocolectomy is necessary, ileal pouch-anal anastomosis (IPAA) is not totally contraindicated, but a staged procedure is strongly recommended. Since improper surgical management of even relatively simple problems, such as haemorrhoids and anal fissure, may affect anal sphincter mechanism and the possibility of performing an adequate ileal-anal anastomosis, the treatment should be as conservative as possible. If necessary, surgery should be performed by a colorectal surgeon aware of IPAA procedure (see Chap. 14 on surgery for UC) [12].

References

1. De Dombal FT, Watts JM, Watkinson G et al (1966) Incidence and management of anorectal abscess, fistula, and fissure in patients with ulcerative colitis. Dis Colon Rectum 9:201–216
2. Edwards F, Truelove SC (1964) The course and prognosis of ulcerative colitis. Part III complications. Gut 32:1–22
3. Bockus HL, Roth JLA, Buchmann E et al (1956) Life history of non-specific ulcerative colitis. Relation of prognosis to anatomical and clinical varieties. Gastroenterologia 86:549–581
4. Fuzy PZ (1961) Surgical management of anorectal complications of chronic ulcerative colitis. South Med J 54:785–817
5. Jackman RJ (1954) Management of anorectal complications of chronic ulcerative colitis. Arch Intern Med 94:420–424

6. Bargen JA (1929) Complications and sequelae of chronic ulcerative colitis. Ann Intern Med 3:335–352

7. Hightower NC, Broders C, Haines RD et al (1958) Chronic ulcerative colitis. II. complications. Am J Dig Dis 3:861–876

8. Waugh JM, Peck D, Lockhart-Mummery HE et al (1960) Crohn's disease (regional enteritis) of the large intestine and its distinction from ulcerative colitis. Gut 1:87–105

9. Lockhart-Mummery HE, Morson BC (1964) Crohn's disease of the large intestine. Gut 5:493–509

10. Price AB (1978) Overlap in the spectrum of non-specific inflammatory bowel disease: "colitis indeterminate". J Clin Pathol 31:567–577

11. Rudolph WG, Uthoff SM, McAuliffe TL et al (2002) Indeterminate colitis. The real story. Dis Colon Rectum 45:1528–1534

12. Hamzaoglu I, Hodin RA (2005) Perianal problems in patients with ulcerative colitis. Inflamm Bowel Dis 11:856–859

13. Zabana Y, Van Domselaar M, Garcia-Planella E et al (2011) Perianal disease in patients with ulcerative colitis: a case-control study. J Crohns Colitis 5:338–341

14. Van Assche G, Dignas A, Bokemeyer B et al (2013) Second European evidence-based consensus on the diagnosis and management of ulcerative colitis: special situations. J Crohns Colitis 7:1–33

15. Van Assche G, Dignass A, Reinisch W et al (2010) The second European evidence-based consensus on the diagnosis and management of Crohn's disease: special situations. J Crohns Colitis 4(1):63–101

16. Parks AG, Gordon PH, Hardcastle J (1976) A classification of fistulain-ano. Br J Surg 63:1–12

17. Katsanos K, Ignatiadou E, Sarandi M et al (2010) Fournier's gangrene complicating ulcerative colitis. J Crohns colitis 4:203–206

Imaging of Perianal Inflammatory Disorders in Ulcerative Colitis

13

Chiara Villa

13.1 Perianal Disease in Ulcerative Colitis Patients

Perianal disease (PAD) associated with ulcerative colitis (UC) was initially described nearly six decades ago, and many reports have documented a high prevalence of such problems in patients with UC. Early studies suggested that the rate of perianal complications in patients with UC was in the range of 20–25 % [1, 2]. These high reported rates of perianal problems in UC were misleading, because colonic Crohn's disease (CD) was first recognized only in the early 1960s and proper descriptions of indeterminate colitis (IC) occurred in the late 1970s; many patients thought in the past to have UC and perianal disease really had either CD or IC [1]. In addition, most references of PAD in UC were published before the widespread use of endoscopy for the diagnosis of these diseases [3].

Currently, there is consensus about the fact that perianal disease sometimes complicates true UC with an incidence approaching 5 %, most often as a haemorrhoids and fissures, and occasionally as fistulas and abscesses [3, 4].

In clinical practice, diagnosis of perianal complications in a UC patient should raise the suspicion of a misdiagnosed colonic CD and re-evaluation of clinical, endoscopic, histological and imaging findings is suggested, knowing that PAD can be present in up to 26 % of CD patients [3, 4].

Zabana et al. in a case-control study involving 758 UC patients demonstrated that the majority of the patients (70 %) who developed PAD did not meet diagnostic criteria of CD, despite diagnostic reassessment [3].

On the other hand, little is known about PAD among true UC patients. Suppurative perianal lesions are strongly associated with active UC and distal or extensive colonic involvement [3, 4]. The pathogenesis is probably multifactorial, involving an immunocompromised state, diarrhoea causing alterations of the anal crypts and possible transmural progression of mucosal abnormalities in severe forms of UC [1, 4].

Fever, bleeding or purulent discharge in UC patients should not be clinically underestimated and attributed to a colonic disease relapse, possibly leading to inappropriate treatment. Although perianal problems are rarely life-threatening, they are often associated with prolonged discomfort, chronic ill health and diminished quality of life. Unrecognized perianal suppuration in patients with UC can result in dangerous conditions such as Fournier's gangrene and sepsis, particularly in diabetic patients and in those patients taking immunosuppressive drugs. Moreover, PAD in UC patients who undergo colectomy is associated with high complication rates after ileal pouch anal anastomosis (IPAA) [1]. In fact, it is demonstrated that these

C. Villa (✉)
Radiology Department, 'Luigi Sacco' University Hospital, via G.B. Grassi 74, 20157 Milan, Italy
e-mail: chiara.villa@hotmail.it

M. Tonolini (ed.), *Imaging of Ulcerative Colitis*,
DOI: 10.1007/978-88-470-5409-7_13, © Springer-Verlag Italia 2014

patients are more prone to anastomotic leaks and other complications after IPAA and that improper surgical management of perianal fistulas may affect the anal sphincter mechanism, leading to poor functional outcomes after IPAA [5–7].

13.2 Perianal Disease in Patients After IPAA Surgery

Although restorative proctocolectomy with IPAA has become the surgical treatment of choice for patients with refractory UC or UC with dysplasia, surgical, inflammatory and non-inflammatory adverse sequelae are common, leading to pouch excision or permanent diversion in 4–10 % of cases [8–14]. Pouchitis, a non-specific inflammation of the ileal reservoir, is the most common long-term complication in patients with IPAA, recurring in more than 50 % patients [14]. Other pouch-related complications can occur, and they include strictures, perianal fistulas and perianal abscesses; the overall incidence rates of these complications are 12–22 % [10]. Many of these complications may be associated to de novo CD of the pouch, a specific clinical condition which may develop weeks to years after IPAA for UC with reported cumulative frequencies ranging from 2.7 to 13 % [8, 9]. The aetiology and pathogenesis of CD of the pouch are not clear. It has been postulated that IPAA with components of procedure-associated ischaemia, anastomosis and faecal stasis may create a CD-friendly environment [9].

In patients with IPAA, fistulas can originate at any level of the pouch and extend into any adjacent hollow organs or to the skin. Based on the cause, pouch fistulas can be classified into pouch CD-related fistulas or non-pouch CD-related fistulas, and their treatment is different [8].

A fistula at the pouch-anal anastomosis level is usually a later presentation of initial anastomotic leak, and it can track to various adjacent locations such as the prostate, urethra, vagina, gluteal muscle space or skin [8]. Immediate post-operative pelvic sepsis occurs in 5–20 % of patients, and it is associated with fistulas in

25 % of patients [8]. Nevertheless, in clinical practice, a persistent anastomotic fistula without history of initial anastomotic leak, particularly when it develops more than 6–12 months after ileostomy takedown, should raise the suspicion of CD [8].

Fistulas below the anastomosis level can result from CD of the pouch or cryptoglandar sepsis. Cryptoglandar sepsis occurs in patients with underlying UC with late spontaneous development of fistula, which sometimes is difficult to distinguish from CD [8]. Recurrent, multiple, complex or anovaginal features of fistulas would suggest a diagnosis of CD, especially if other perianal lesions exist [8].

Pouch-vaginal fistulas (PVF) are a unique yet common condition with IPAA, a major source of morbidity and one of the most common causes for pouch failure [8, 9]. The incidence rate of ileal pouch-vaginal fistulas is 4–12 % [10]. A variety of factors have been implicated in the development of PVF, including failure to exclude CD preoperatively, post-operative pelvic sepsis, anastomotic leak, separation or stricture of anastomosis, postoperative CD of the pouch, cryptoglandular inflammation and incorporation of the posterior vaginal wall during stapled anastomosis [8, 9]. PVF can develop early (<6 months after IPAA) or late (>12 months after IPAA). PVF can present at, below or above the anastomosis and presents as a simple or complex fistula with multiple fistulous tracts [8]. Also in this case, a diagnosis of CD should always be suspected, especially if PVF develops late, is complex and outside the pouch-anal anastomosis [8, 9]. PVF can persist even though repeated surgical attempts for closure are performed; the success rate of surgical treatment of PVF is approximately 50 % in patients with an initial failure of surgery [10].

13.3 Imaging of Perianal Disease

Imaging of perianal space is crucial for a prompt diagnosis and an accurate assessment of PAD in UC patients, especially for those potential candidates for surgery, both in pre- and post-operative periods.

Nowadays, *magnetic resonance imaging (MRI)* is considered the gold standard technique in the evaluation of PAD, due to its multiplanarity and high soft-tissue contrast resolution [15, 16]. It has been demonstrated that MRI is highly accurate, with sensitivity and specificity, respectively, of 100 and 86 % in detection of fistulas primary tracts, and respectively, of 96 and 97 % in detection of abscesses [17]. In particular, MRI is the examination of choice to study complex perianal fistulas, being able to detect sepsis outside the anal sphincter and its relationship with the sphincter and levator ani muscles [18]. Besides an accurate morphological evaluation of the perianal space, contrast-enhanced MRI provides information about perianal disease activity and may be helpful in differentiating active sepsis from fibrosis (Fig. 13.2) [19–22]. Finally, the lack of irradiation and limited biologic invasiveness of gadolinium contrast are particularly beneficial in young patients with chronic inflammatory bowel diseases, who often need imaging follow-up studies [23].

Recently, pelvic MRI has been reported as a very accurate modality for the assessment of post-operative IPAA anatomy and possible complications, and it is well tolerated even by patients with anal pain or stenosis [23]. The normal ileal pouch reservoir is identified by the small hypointense ferromagnetic artefacts (signal voids) on all sequences, corresponding to the location of the metallic staples; fistulizing complications and abscesses show the same features as in UC and CD non-treated patients (Fig. 13.3) [23]. MRI has also proved to be particularly valuable in the differentiation of pouch-related pelvic sepsis, even in patients with normal endoscopic findings, from simple pouchitis [23].

At our centre a standardized protocol for perianal MRI examination is performed, in order to maximize reproducibility and help the comparison during follow-up studies. Images are acquired with external phased-array coil without special bowel preparation.

Sagittal-oriented T2-weighted turbo-or fast-spin echo (TSE/FSE) sequences are initially used to obtain a panoramic view of both the urogenital structures and the anorectal tract, and to allow a precise planning of the subsequent axial and coronal sequences, which must be oriented along oblique planes perpendicularly and parallel to the longitudinal axis of the anal canal, respectively [24]. Axial and coronal T2-weighted images are essential for the differentiation of the internal and external anal sphincter components, and provide the intrinsic soft-tissue contrast needed to identify fistulas and abscesses which show hyperintense signal and scar tissue which show hypointense signal [24]. T1-weighted coronal images are suitable to identify the levator ani and thus to differentiate between the supralevator, ischiorectal and ischioanal spaces [24].

Axial and coronal fat-saturated T2-weighted sequences are used to increase the conspicuity of fluid-containing tracks or abscesses; fluid, pus and granulation tissue are seen as areas of high signal intensity on a background of low-signal-intensity fat (Fig. 13.4) [25]. T1-weighted fat saturated sequences may be useful in the post-operative setting to identify recent haemorrhage [24]. Intravenous paramagnetic gadolinium-based contrast is routinely administered and axial and coronal T1-weighted sequences are acquired, with fat saturation in at least one plane. These sequences greatly help visual recognition of active disease, since inflamed granulation tissue in the walls of abscesses and fistulas enhances, whereas chronic fistulas usually do not, and fluid in tracts and the contents of purulent abscesses remain T1-hypointense (Fig. 13.5) [24]. A recent study demonstrated a significant association between the increase in the signal intensity of the fistula after contrast administration and the severity of perianal disease, proposing a diagnostic tool to assess disease activity [22].

Anal fistulas are classified according to their progression relative to the anal sphincter and pelvic floor structures [25]. To locate the point of origin and describe the direction of the fistulous track, the surgical "anal clock" scheme is currently used, which corresponds exactly with the view of the anal canal on axial MR images obtained with the patient in the supine decubitus position (anterior perineum located at 12 o'clock, natal cleft at 6 o'clock, left lateral aspect of the anal canal at 3 o'clock and right lateral aspect at 9 o'clock) [25].

There are two main classification systems for perianal fistulas, based on the relationship between the primary track and the anal sphincter muscles: the Parks classification and the St James's University Hospital classification [25].

Relying on surgical findings, Parks et al. described perianal fistulas in the coronal plane according to the course of the fistula and its relationships to the internal and external sphincters [26]. Fistulas were classified into four groups: intersphincteric, transsphincteric, suprasphincteric and extrasphincteric, as shown in Fig. 13.1 [27].

The St James's University Hospital classification was proposed by radiologists on the basis of imaging findings and related the Parks surgical classification to anatomic MR imaging findings in the axial and coronal planes [28]. It uses anatomic landmarks in the axial plane familiar to radiologists and considers the primary fistulous track as well as secondary extensions and abscesses in evaluating and classifying fistulas. The classification grades

fistulas into five groups: Grade 1, simple linear intersphincteric fistula; Grade 2, intersphincteric with abscess or secondary track; Grade 3, transsphincteric; Grade 4, transsphincteric with abscess or secondary track in ischiorectal or ischioanal fossa; Grade 5, supralevator and translevator [25].

The role of *computed tomography (CT)* in the evaluation of PAD is limited because CT, exposing patients to significant amounts of ionizing radiations, is not suitable for follow-up. Conversely, in emergency settings CT examinations are widely requested to investigate acute abdominal/perianal pain in UC patients, and to assess clinically suspected complications during the early post-operative period in patients undergoing IPAA. Since current fast multidetector scanners allow a panoramic coverage of the entire abdomen and pelvis in a few seconds and provide isotropic image reconstructions on arbitrary planes, longer coverage including the perianal region is suggested when examining acute UC patients. Intravenous iodinated contrast medium is usually injected unless contraindicated [23, 29].

Perianal abscesses and fistulas that are filled by air or fluid can be identified on CT because of adequate contrast between their hypodense contents and the enhancing, inflamed granulation tissue present in the walls (Fig. 13.6) [29].

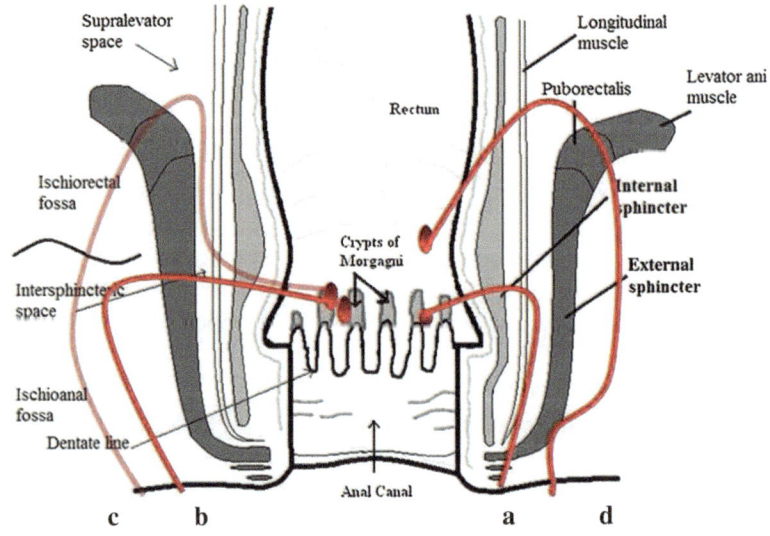

Fig. 13.1 The Parks classification of perianal fistulas. *a* Intersphincteric fistula, *b* transsphincteric fistula, *c* suprasphincteric fistula, *d* extrasphincteric (translevator) fistula (Reprinted with permission from reference no. [27])

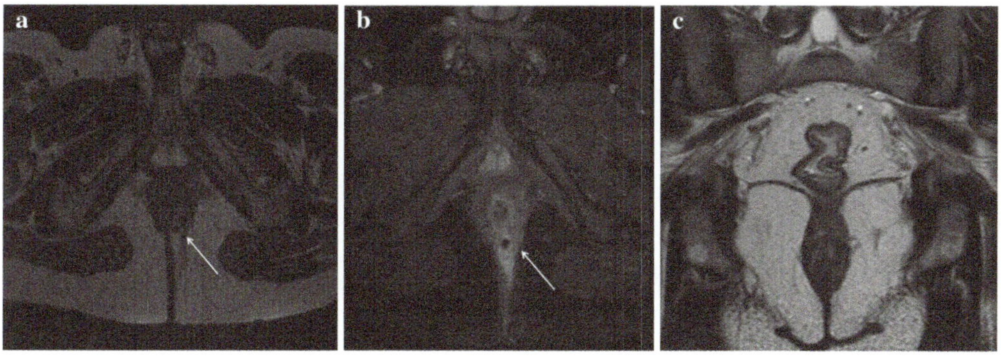

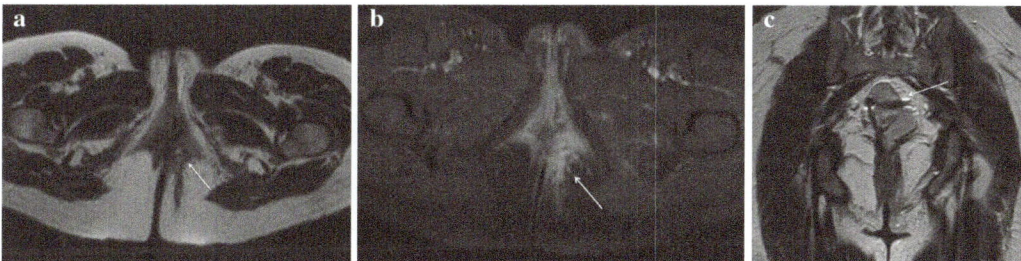

Fig. 13.2 Male patient with active UC and evidence of purulent perianal discharge. **a** On MRI axial T2-weighted sequences, a small simple transsphincteric hyperintense fistulous tract was detected at 5 o'clock. **b** T1-weighted fat saturated axial sequences after intravenous contrast administration showed vivid enhancement of the fistula and a better visualization of a tiny hypointense air bubble within the lumen. **c** In the same examination, T2-weighted coronal sequences imaged the rectum which presented thickened and hyperintense walls indicating active inflammation

Fig. 13.3 Female patient with IPAA complaining of perianal pain. **a** On MRI axial T2-weighted sequences a complex transsphincteric hyperintense fistulous tract was detected at 3 o'clock. **b** T1-weighted fat saturated axial sequences after intravenous contrast administration showed vivid enhancement of the fistula and allowed to depict its small multiple ramifications. **c** In the same examination, T2-weighted coronal sequences offered an optimal view of the ileal pouch reservoir identified by hypointense ferromagnetic artifacts (signal voids), the anal canal and levator ani muscles, and the fistulous primary track in left ischioanal fossa (Reprinted with permission from reference no. [38])

CT is accurate in detecting perianal abscesses, and the involvement at the level of or above the levator ani muscles is identifiable on coronal images [29]. However, intrinsic CT contrast resolution limits the differentiation between different soft-tissue structures such as the pelvic muscles, active inflammatory changes and fibrotic scar tissue and CT does not have sufficient accuracy to correctly classify fistulas. Inhomogeneity, abnormal density or enhancement involving the ischioanal fat spaces indicate the presence of transsphincteric inflammation to be further investigated with MRI [29, 30].

CT is reliable in the diagnosis of pouch-related septic complications, suggested by the detection of extraluminal air, fluid or contrast material [23]. At CT, the ileal pouch reservoir is identified as a fluid-filled structure in the anatomical location of the resected rectum, with metallic surgical staples located 180° to each other. The pouch-anal anastomosis, indicated by the presence of hyperdense clips, should also be identified as it represents a possible source of leakage. In order to rule out early anastomotic leakage after IPAA surgery, bowel opacification with water-soluble contrast per os or per rectum may be useful [23].

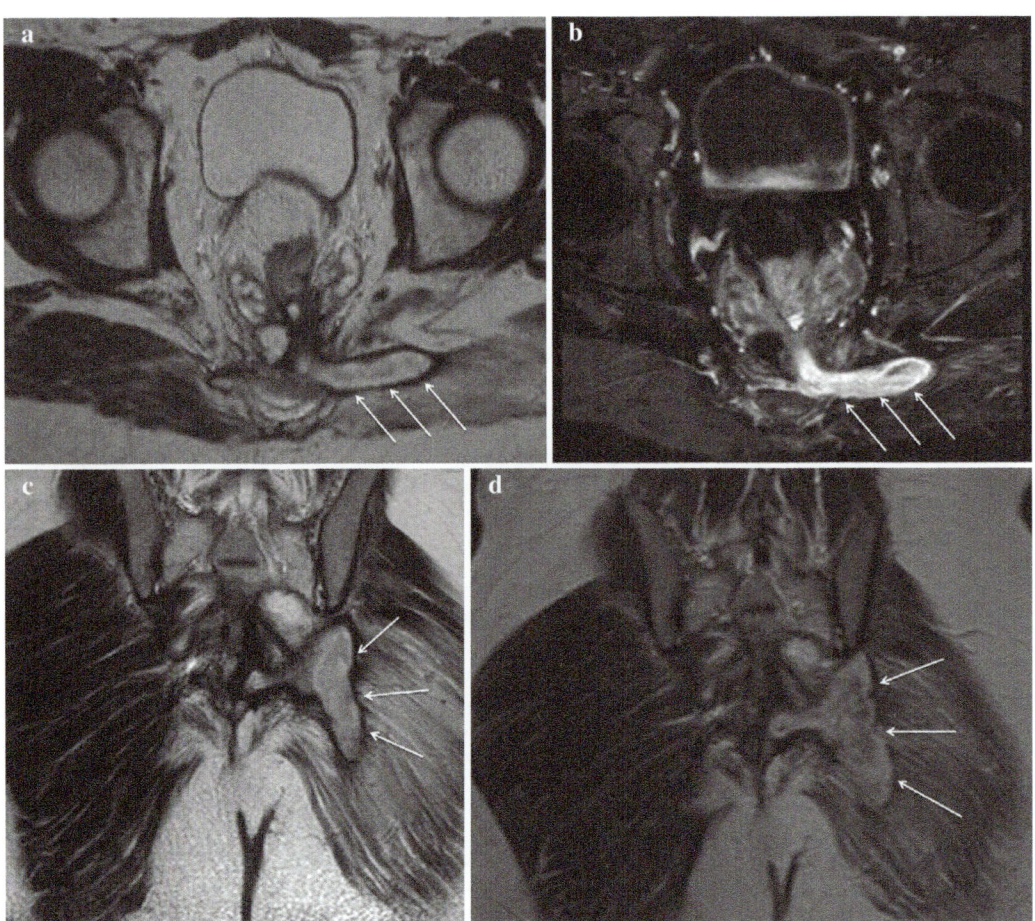

Fig. 13.4 Male patient after proctocolectomy with IPAA complaining of perianal pain and massive purulent perineal discharge. **a** MRI T2-weighted axial sequences showed a large hyperintense fistula originating from the pouch-anal anastomosis level at 6 o'clock directed toward the *left* gluteal muscle. **b** On T1-weighted fat saturated axial sequences after intravenous contrast administration the large fistulous track strongly enhanced because of the presence of granulation tissue, confirming active inflammation. **c** T2-weighted coronal sequences best depicted the extent of the fistula in the posterior perineum and documented the involvement of *left* gluteal muscle which presented hyperintense signal suggestive of oedema. **d** On post-contrast T1-weighted coronal sequences the fistula showed diffuse enhancement

Other imaging modalities currently used in the evaluation and follow-up of PAD are *transanal and transperineal ultrasound* which are easy to perform, low cost, ionizing radiation free and accurate in detecting perianal fistulas and abscesses with results comparable to pelvic MRI [30–34].

Transanal ultrasound, performed using a high-frequency rotating endoprobe, can accurately assess and classify perianal complications of UC, whether spontaneously occurring or complicating IPAA, providing at the same time a sonographic assessment of the rectal wall [31].

Perineal ultrasound, performed using high-frequency curved microconvex and linear-array probes, assesses fistulous and sinus tracts as well as abscesses and collections, documenting their relationship with the anal canal, the scrotum in men, and the labia and vagina in women [31]. In particular, perineal ultrasound is useful to detect perianal fistulas and inflammatory tissue or masses located outside the field of view of

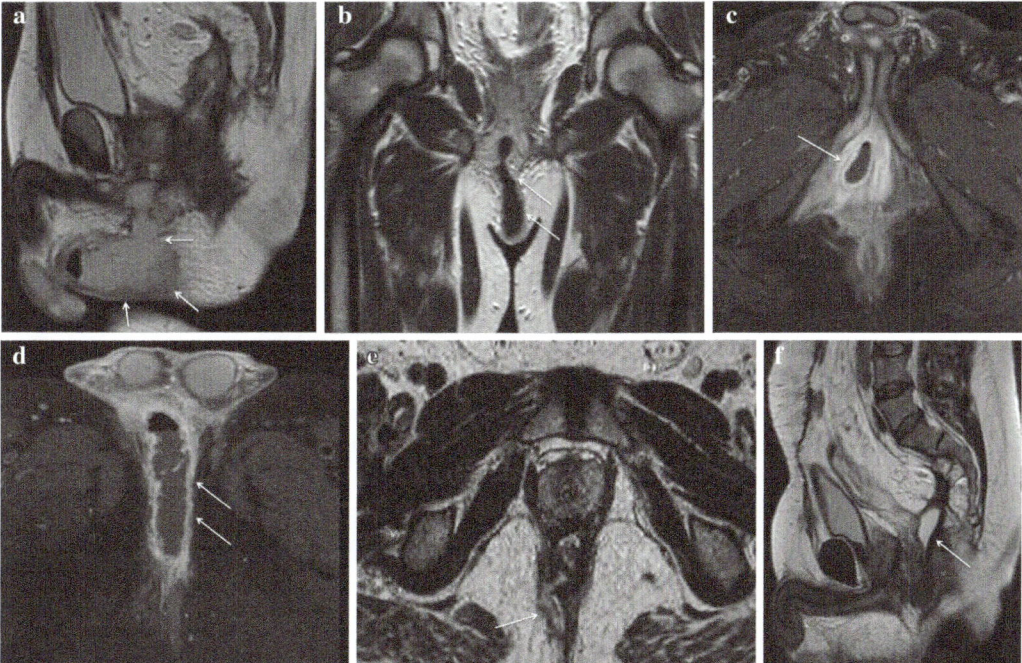

Fig. 13.5 Male patient with IPAA, fever and strong perianal and genital pain. **a** On MRI T2-weighted sagittal sequences a bulky hyperintense fluid collection was detected in the anterior perineum, extending toward the scrotum. **b** T1-weighted coronal sequences after intravenous contrast administration best depicted a large fistulous track originating from the pouch-anal anastomosis level between 6 and 7 o'clock. Inflamed granulation tissue in the walls of the fistula presented bright signal, whereas fluid in the lumen remained T1-hypointense. **c, d** Post-contrast T1-weighted fat saturated axial sequences highlighted the presence of a large abscess in the *right* anterior perineum on the way of the transsphincteric fistula involving the crus of the penis and the scrotum. The collection showed typical enhancing walls, purulent hypointense content and a tiny fluid-air level. **e, f** MRI performed on the same patient after surgical drainage of the abscess. T2-weighted axial sequences (**e**) assessed a satisfactory outcome of the procedure: only a small fistolous track remained. In the same examination, T2-weighted sagittal sequences (**f**) better portrayed the complete surgical abscess drainage in the anterior perineum, but pointed out the occurrence of a hyperintense fluid collection posterior to the pouch-anal anastomotic site in the presacral space indicative of a sinus (Reprinted with permission from reference no. [38])

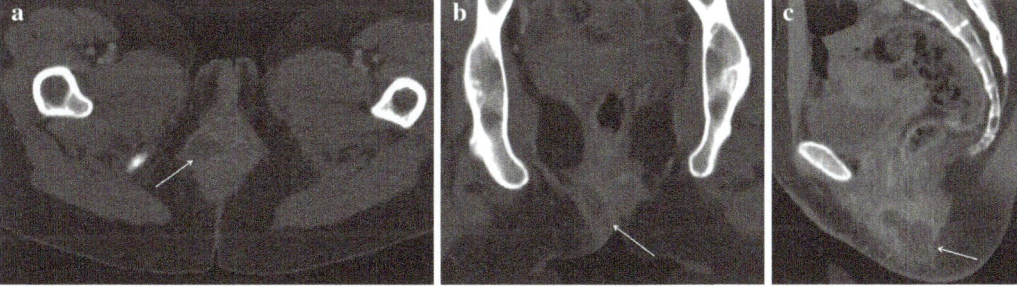

Fig. 13.6 Female patient with active UC and fever, complaining of pain in perianal region. **a** In an emergency setting, CT detected a large perianal abscess with hypodense contents and enhancing walls in the intersphincteric space extending in the *right* ischioanal fossa. **b** Coronal reformations showed that the abscess did not cross the levator ani muscle and was limited to perianal space. **c** Sagittal reformations showed the real extent of the abscess and the involvement of the ipsilateral gluteus

transanal ultrasound, or when the latter examination cannot be performed in a patient with severe anal pain or stricture [31].

Fistula tracts and abscesses complicating UC resemble those of Crohn's disease. Fistulous tracts may be described as hypoechoic, round to oval structures in an intersphincteric location, sometimes with internal hyperechoic echoes as a result of gas or air within an abscess or a fistulous tract [31]. An opening within the mucosa of the anal canal or within the rectum may identified as a gap or disruption of the integrity of the echo structure of the normal wall [31]. An abscess may be detected sonographically as a mass which is either anechoic (without internal echoes) or hypoechoic (with internal echoes secondary to cellular debris) [30].

The limits of these techniques are the dependency on the expertise of the operators and on the availability of the necessary diagnostic tools.

13.4 Imaging of Genital Tract Involvement

Anovaginal, rectovaginal and pouch-vaginal fistulas are usually diagnosed on the basis of typical clinical symptoms such as recurrent vaginal infections, air, enteric or fecal vaginal discharge and a gynecologic or surgical examination under anesthesia.

In the past, fistulography and water-soluble contrast rectal enema were routinely used to study anovaginal fistulas. Nowadays transrectal and transperineal ultrasound are used as initial non-invasive examinations [35].

Anovaginal fistulas can be depicted also with phased-array coil or endoanal MRI. Previous studies assessed that MR imaging with phased-array coil may identify most of the larger fistulous tracts, whereas endoluminal MRI thanks to its higher spatial resolution provides a better visualization of rectovaginal septum and vagina, allowing the detection of smaller tracts [36]. However, for a comprehensive evaluation of perianal disease, the use of a phased-array coil should be preferred because it offers a larger field of view covering the entire pelvis and avoids the use of endoluminal coil, which is always badly tolerated by patients with active PAD. The sagittal plane is considered the most reliable plane for visualization of the fistula (Fig. 13.7) [36, 37].

Simple vaginal fistulas, consisting of thin fluid-filled tracks lined by granulation tissue, may be identified as T2-hyperintense linear structures originating from the ventral aspect of

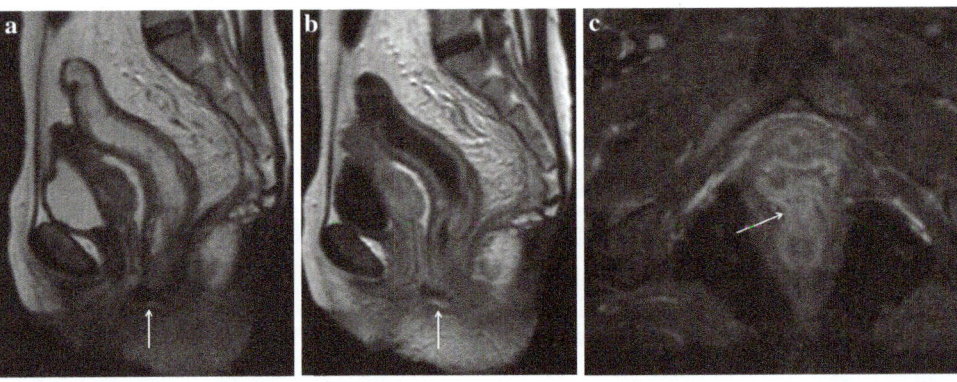

Fig. 13.7 Female patient with IPAA suffering from recurrent pouchitis, air and faecal vaginal discharge. **a** On MRI T2-weighted sagittal sequences a short thick fistulous track between the anal canal and the vagina below the anastomosis level was detected; it was strongly hypointense suggesting the presence of air within the lumen. On the same sequences, pouch walls appeared thickened and hyperintense indicating active inflammation. **b** T1-weighted sagittal sequences after intravenous contrast administration demonstrated strong enhancement of both fistulas and pouch walls. **c** Post-contrast T1-weighted fat-saturated axial sequences better defined the location of the fistula at 12 o'clock and vaginal walls involvement. The granulation tissue within the fistolous track showed diffuse enhancement

the anal canal, which shows contrast-enhancement on T1 fat-saturated sequences. Abscess collections occupying the anovaginal septum are very easily detected as fluid-like, non-enhancing collections, with peripheral rim enhancement after intravenous contrast [35].

In our still unpublished experience, the sensitivity of MRI with phased array coil in the detection of anovaginal fistulas approached 50 %, since only the largest fistulas and/or fistulas with associated septal abscesses were correctly identified. Smaller simple fistulas were often invisible on MRI.

Nevertheless, non-specific inflammatory changes involving the vulvar/vaginal region or the rectovaginal septum, characterized by a diffuse T2-weighted hyperintense signal and positive contrast enhancement should be considered suspicious as indirect signs of the presence of anogenital fistulas in symptomatic patients. As well as reported in association with CD, male patients may suffer from genital involvement,

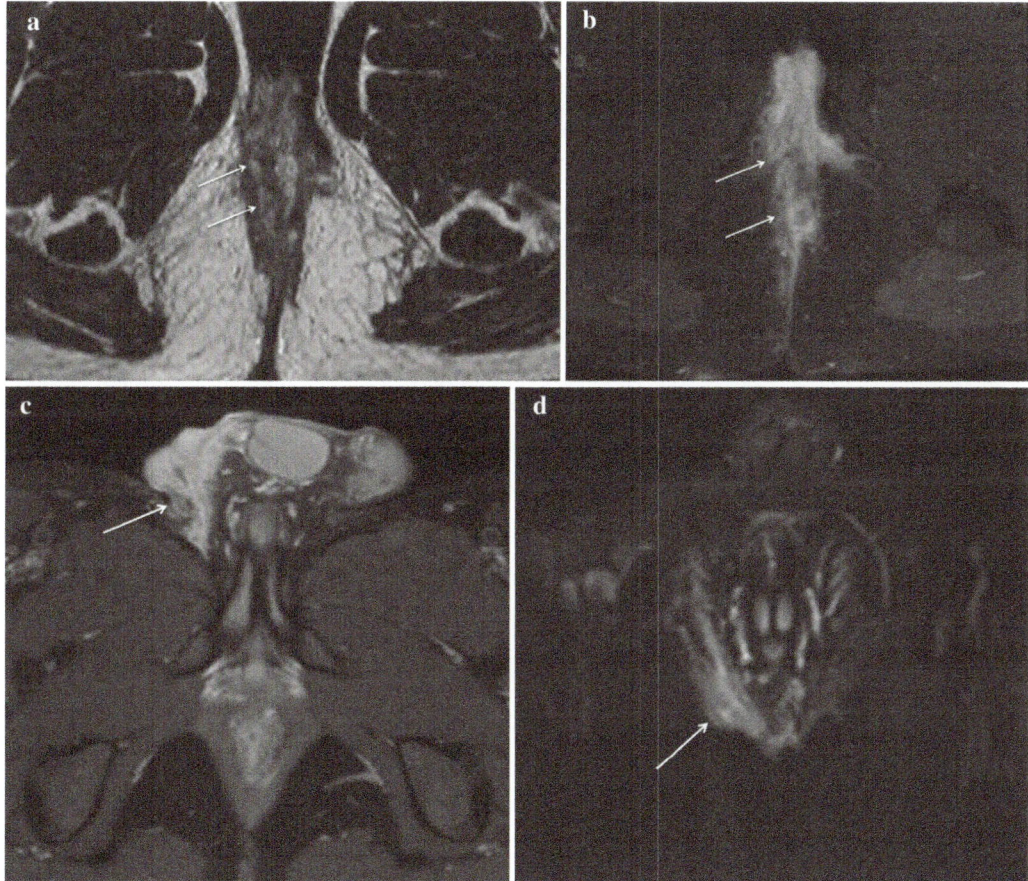

Fig. 13.8 Male patient with UC suffering from perianal pain with suspected hydrocele. **a** T2-weighted axial sequences confirmed the presence of fluid small hyperintense collections extending from the anal canal to the crus of the penis. These findings were considered as an indirect sign of the extension of a perianal inflammatory disease to the genital region, even if MRI was not able to identify the primary fistulous track in this case. **b**, **c** T1-weighted fat-saturated axial sequences after intravenous contrast administration documented an intense scattered enhancement of the anterior perineum and the crus of the penis suggestive of active inflammation. Enhancing hyperintense tissue was detectable also within the *right* portion of the scrotum which was enlarged. **d** T2-weighted fat-saturated coronal sequences best imaged the involvement of the scrotum with hyperintense signal on the *right* side confirming the presence of inflammatory tissue and fluid

including prostate, scrotum and proximal urethra abscesses, usually originated from direct extension of perianal inflammatory disease. MRI easily detects these abnormalities as fluid-filled, peripherally enhancing structures usually associated with perianal fistulas (Fig. 13.8) [35].

References

1. Hamzaoglu I, Hodin RA (2005) Perianal problems in patients with ulcerative colitis. Inflamm Bowel Dis 11:856–859
2. de Dombal FT, Watts JM, Watkinson G et al (1966) Incidence and management of anorectal abscess, fistula, and fissure in patients with ulcerative colitis. Dis Colon Rectum 9:201–216
3. Zabana Y, Van Domselaar M, Garcia-Planella E et al (2011) Perianal disease in patients with ulcerative colitis: a case-control study. J Crohn's Colitis 5:338–341
4. Tonolini M, Bareggi E (2011, Jul 21) Unusual perianal inflammatory disease complicating ulcerative colitis. http://www.eurorad.org/case.php?id=9119
5. Richard CS, Cohen Z, Stern HS et al (1997) Outcome of the pelvic pouch procedure in patients with prior perianal disease. Dis Colon Rectum 40:647–652
6. Alexander F, Sarigol S, DiFiore J et al (2003) Fate of the pouch in 151 pediatric patients after ileal pouch anastomosis. J Pediatr Surg 38:78–82
7. Fazio VW, Tekkis PP, Remzi F et al (2003) Quantification of risk for pouch failure after ileal pouch anal anastomosis surgery. Ann Surg 238:605–617
8. Shen B, Remzi FH, Lavery IC et al (2008) A proposed classification of ileal pouch disorders and associated complications after restorative proctocolectomy. Clin Gastroenterol Hepatol 6(2):145–158
9. Shen B (2010) Diagnosis and management of postoperative ileal pouch disorders. Clin Colon Rectal Surg 23:259–268
10. Baik SH, Kim WH (2012) A comprehensive review of inflammatory bowel disease focusing on surgical management. J Korean Soc Coloproctol 28(3):121–131
11. Goldstein NS, Sanford WW, Bodzin JH (1997) Crohn's-like complications in patients with ulcerative colitis after total proctocolectomy and ileal pouch-anal anastomosis. Am J Surg Pathol 21:1343–1353
12. Viscido A, Habib FI, Kohn A et al (2003) Infliximab in refractory pouchitis complicated by fistulae following ileo-anal pouch for ulcerative colitis. Aliment Pharmacol Ther 17:1263–1271
13. Beliard A, Prudhomme M (2010) Ileal reservoir with ileo-anal anastomosis: long-term complications. J Visc Surg 147(3):137–144
14. Van Assche G, Dignass A, Bokemeyer B et al (2013) Second European evidence-based consensus on the diagnosis and management of ulcerative colitis part 3: special situations. J Crohn's Colitis 7:1–33
15. Morris J, Spencer JA, Ambrose NS (2000) MR imaging classification of perianal fistulas and its implications for patients management. Radiographics 20:623–637
16. Halligan S, Stoker J (2006) Imaging of fistula in ano. Radiology 239:18–33
17. Beets-Tan RG, Beets GL, van der Hoop AG et al (2001) Preoperative MR imaging of anal fistulas: does it really help the surgeon? Radiology 218:75–84
18. Sahni VA, Ahmad R, Burling D (2008) Which method is best for imaging of perianal fistula? Abdom Imaging 33:26–30
19. Van Assche G, Vanbeckevoort D, Bielen D et al (2003) Magnetic resonance imaging of the effects of infliximab on perianal fistulizing Crohn's disease. Am J Gastroenterol 98:332–339
20. Bell SJ, Halligan S, Windsor AC et al (2003) Response of fistulating Crohn's disease to infliximab treatment assessed by magnetic resonance imaging. Aliment Pharmacol Ther 17:387–393
21. Spencer JA, Ward J, Beckingham IJ et al (1996) Dynamic contrast-enhanced MR imaging of perianal fistulas. AJR 167:735–741
22. Villa C, Pompili G, Franceschelli G et al (2012) Role of magnetic resonance imaging in evaluation of the activity of perianal Crohn's disease. Eur J Radiol 81:616–622
23. Tonolini M (2012) Ulcerative colits and ileal pouch surgery. In: Tonolini M, Maconi G (eds) Imaging of perianal inflammatory diseases. Springer, Milan, pp 177–183
24. Campari A, Tonolini M (2012) MRI study protocol. In: Tonolini M, Maconi G (eds) Imaging of perianal inflammatory diseases. Springer, Milan, pp 127–132
25. Criado JM, del Salto JG, Rivas P et al (2012) MR imaging evaluation of perianal fistulas: spectrum of imaging features. RadioGraphics 32:175–194
26. Parks AG, Gordon PH, Hardcastle JD (1976) A classification of fistula-in-ano. Br J Surg 63(1):1–12
27. Maccioni F, bella G, Buonocore V (2012) Perianal Crohn's disease MRI classification and staging. In: Tonolini M, Maconi G (eds) Imaging of perianal inflammatory diseases. Springer, Milan, pp 143–164
28. Morris J, Spencer JA, Ambrose NS (2000) MR imaging classification of perianal fistulas and its implications for patient management. RadioGraphics 20(3):623–637
29. Norsa AH, Tonolini M (2012) Techniques and role of CT in perianal disease. In: Tonolini M, Maconi G (eds) Imaging of perianal inflammatory diseases. Springer, Milan, pp 213–218

30. Ardizzone S, Maconi G, Cassinotti A (2007) Imaging of perianal Crohn's disease. Dig Liver Dis 39:970–978

31. Maconi G, Furfaro F, Bezzio C (2012) Ulcerative colitis. In: Tonolini M, Maconi G (eds) Imaging of perianal inflammatory diseases. Springer, Milan, pp 95–102

32. Schwartz DA, Wiersema MJ, Dudiak KM et al (2001) A comparison of endoscopic ultrasound, magnetic resonance imaging, and exam under anesthesia for evaluation of Crohn's perianal fistulas. Gastroenterology 121:1064–1072

33. Wedemeyer J, Kirchhoff T, Sellge G et al (2004) Transcutaneous perianal sonography: a sensitive method for the detection of perianal inflammatory lesions in Crohn's disease. World J Gastroenterol 10:2859–2863

34. Maconi G, Ardizzone S, Greco S et al (2007) Transperineal ultrasound in the detection of perianal and rectovaginal fistulae in Crohn's disease. Am J Gastroenterol 102(10):2214–2219

35. Tonolini M, Villa C, Campari A et al (2013) Common and unusual urogenital Crohn's disease complications: spectrum of cross-sectional imaging findings. Abdom Imaging 38:32–41

36. Dwarkasing S, Hussain SM, Hop WCJ et al (2004) Anovaginal fistulas: evaluation with endoanal MR imaging. Radiology 231:123–128

37. Hosseinzadeh K, Heller MT, Houshmand G (2012) Imaging of the female perineum in adults. Radiographics 32:E129–E168

38. Tonolini M, Campari A, Bianco R (2011) Ileal pouch and related complications: spectrum of imaging findings with emphasis on MRI. Abdom Imaging 36:698–706

Ileal Pouch-Anal Anastomosis Surgery: Surgical Techniques

14

Gianluca Matteo Sampietro, Francesco Colombo, Silvia Casiraghi and Diego Foschi

14.1 Introduction

Ulcerative colitis (UC) is an inflammatory bowel disease (IBD) of unknown aetiology arising from an interaction between genetic and environmental factors. UC is a lifelong disease and a curative medical therapy is not yet available. The incidence is highest in the developed countries, and in Europe there is a North to South gradient, but it is increasing also in the Southern and Eastern countries. The incidence of UC is 9–20 cases per 10^5 person-years, and prevalence is from 156–291 per 10^5 cases per people. Most of the patients achieve remission under medical treatment. Systemic steroids are mainly used for induction of remission, while maintenance is based on the use of aminosalicylates compounds for mild disease up to immunosuppressants and biologics for severe disease. Surgery has an incidence of 20–30 % of the cases within 10 years of diagnosis, with the highest rate in the first 2 years of disease onset and in patients with the whole colon involved. Nowadays, surgery is the only curative treatment available for UC. The expanding use of immunosuppressants and anti-TNF-α agents has not decreased the need for surgery. Life expectancy for UC patients is not different from the general population [1, 2].

14.2 Indications for Surgical Treatment

There are several indications for surgery in UC patients, including the failure of or the intolerance to medical therapy, intractable fulminant colitis, toxic megacolon, perforation, uncontrollable bleeding, colonic strictures, growth retardation in children and dysplasia or cancer. From a clinical point of view, these indications should be divided into emergency, urgent and elective.

Emergency settings are due to toxic megacolon (TM), perforation and severe bleeding. Toxic dilation is defined as total or segmental colonic dilation of more than 5.5 cm, without evidence of obstruction and associated with systemic signs of toxicity (Fig. 14.1). In UC patients the lifetime incidence is 1–2.5 %, and it

G. M. Sampietro (✉)
Head of IBD Surgical Unit—Department of Surgery, "Luigi Sacco" University Hospital, Via GB Grassi, 74, 20157 Milan, Italy
e-mail: gianluca.sampietro@unimi.it

F. Colombo
Division of General Surgery—Department of Surgery, "Luigi Sacco" University Hospital, Via GB Grassi, 74, 20157 Milan, Italy
e-mail: colombo.francesco@hsacco.it

S. Casiraghi
Division of General Surgery—Department of Surgery, "Luigi Sacco" University Hospital, Via GB Grassi, 74, 20157 Milan, Italy
e-mail: casiraghisilvia@gmail.com

D. Foschi
Head of the Department of Surgery, "Luigi Sacco" University Hospital, Via GB Grassi, 74, 20157 Milan, Italy
e-mail: diego.foschi@unimi.it

M. Tonolini (ed.), *Imaging of Ulcerative Colitis*,
DOI: 10.1007/978-88-470-5409-7_14, © Springer-Verlag Italia 2014

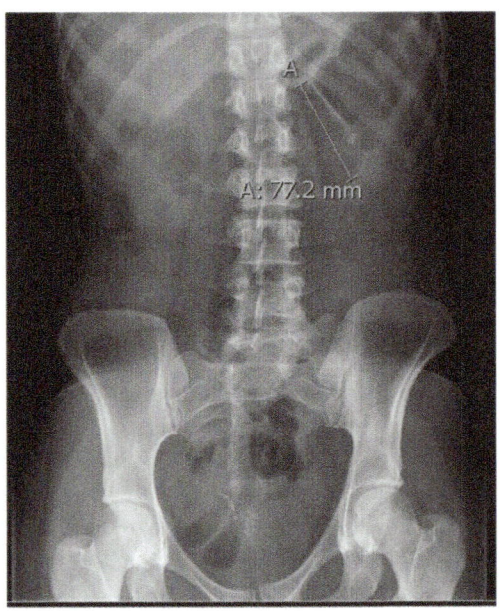

Fig. 14.1 24-year-old female patient presenting toxic dilation of the distal transverse colon before starting rescue medical therapy

accounts for 6 % of all hospital admissions. However, in tertiary IBD centres, up to 17–20 % of admissions present signs and symptoms of toxicity [3]. Perioperative mortality rate is reported to be 6–16 %, but it rises to 27–50 % in case of concomitant perforation. Morbidity rate is 60 %, including a 50 % of severe sepsis and 33 % of postoperative fistulae [4–6]. Perforation accounts for 10 % of surgical emergencies in UC. The incidence is related to the severity and extension of the acute episode, and it should be independent of toxic dilation. The associated mortality rate ranges from 27 to 57 %; the higher the severity and the extension of the attack, the higher the mortality and morbidity rate [7]. Haemorrhage leading to surgery accounts for less than 5 % of emergency procedures. However, 50 % of the patients presenting unmanageable bleeding have concomitant TM, therefore bleeding in a patient with severe acute colitis should always be considered for impending megacolon (Fig. 14.2) [8].

Acute severe colitis accounts for the vast majority of urgent procedures and requires intensive medical treatment; this involves monitoring vital signs, treatment of electrolyte depletion, malnutrition, anaemia and toxicity, which are usually present to some degree. Specific anti-inflammatory treatment with steroids, cyclosporine or anti-TNF-α antibodies can salvage 50 % of the patients, but a high early relapse rate has been reported [8, 9]. In emergency and urgent settings portal vein thrombosis should always be assessed, since it has an incidence of 40 % and a consistent associated morbidity (see dedicated Chap. 9) [10].

Elective surgery is mainly performed for strictures, medical intractability and dysplasia or cancer. Colonic strictures have an incidence of 11 % and should be due to sub-mucosa fibrosis or mucosal hyperplasia. However, biopsies of strictures are often inadequate to role out malignancy and thus patients with long-standing disease, low-grade dysplasia in a symptomatic stricture or a stricture impassable during endoscopy have an indication to surgery. Furthermore, in the presence of a stricture a diagnosis of Crohn's disease (CD) should always be considered for both medical and surgical therapeutic implications [8, 11]. Failure of medical management may be defined as inadequate control of symptoms with intensive medical treatment, chronic disability due to therapy and/or disease, intolerance to any pharmacological compound, medical therapy associated with excessive long-term risk (mainly steroids) and growth failure in the paediatric population [8, 9, 11–13]. Colorectal cancer (CRC) has a cumulative incidence in UC patients of 3.7 %, increasing to 5.4 % in patients with pancolitis. The cancer risk, however, increases over time and it is estimated at 2 % at 10 years, 8 % at 20 years and 18 % at 30 years of disease [14]. While an established diagnosis of CRC is an absolute indication to surgery, the management of dysplasia and dysplasia-associated lesions or masses (DALM) has to be taken with great caution. The European Crohn's and Colitis Organization (ECCO) has published extensive practical parameters on this topic, in dedicated guidelines [15]. In fact, 42 % of patients with high-grade dysplasia and 43 % of patients with DALM may have a synchronous CRC at the time of colectomy [16].

Fig. 14.2 21-year-old male presenting with acute colitis and severe bleeding (*upper left*). *Upper right*, after 36 h of intensive medical treatment the patient presented important dilation of the *right* colon (*arrows*), systemic signs of toxicity and massive bleeding. The patient underwent emergency subtotal colectomy. In the *lower* panel is reported the surgical specimen

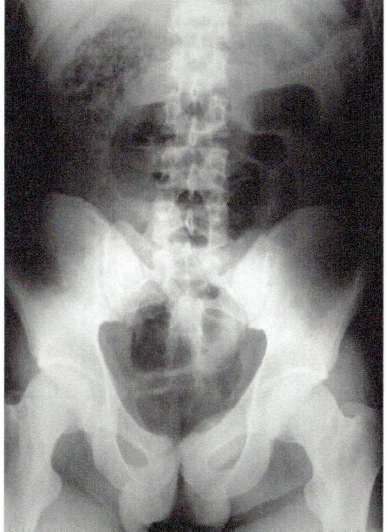
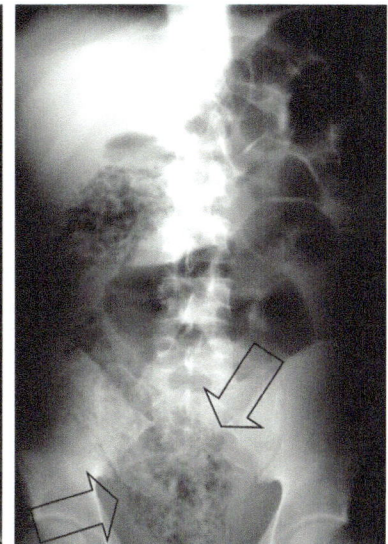

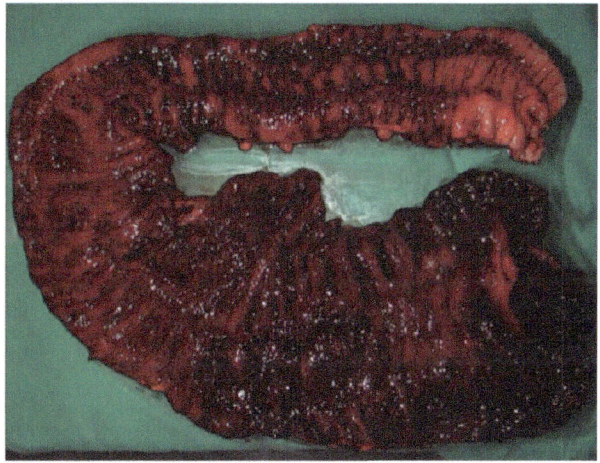

14.3 Surgical Strategy

A number of surgical procedures are available for the treatment of UC, each with its own set of benefits and drawbacks. The surgeon, when planning surgical strategy, has to take into account several factors including patient history (in particular: preoperative medical therapy and previous surgical interventions), medical comorbidities, nutritional status and indication for surgery. The primary goal of surgery for UC is the removal of all diseased colon and rectum with the lowest morbidity and the best quality of life for every single patient. However, accomplishment of this goal may result in a winding

road, and the final decision is dependent on clinical presentation (urgent or elective), anatomical characteristics, patient expectations and requires an on-going dialogue among the patient, the gastroenterologist and the surgeon.

There are four operations available for patients undergoing surgery for UC. These include conventional proctocolectomy with permanent ileostomy or Kock's pouch continent ileostomy, abdominal colectomy with ileo-rectal anastomosis (IRA) and restorative proctocolectomy with ileal-pouch-anal anastomosis (IPAA) (Fig. 14.3).

Total proctocolectomy with end ileostomy has the advantage to be a single procedure that removes all disease and eliminates the risk of

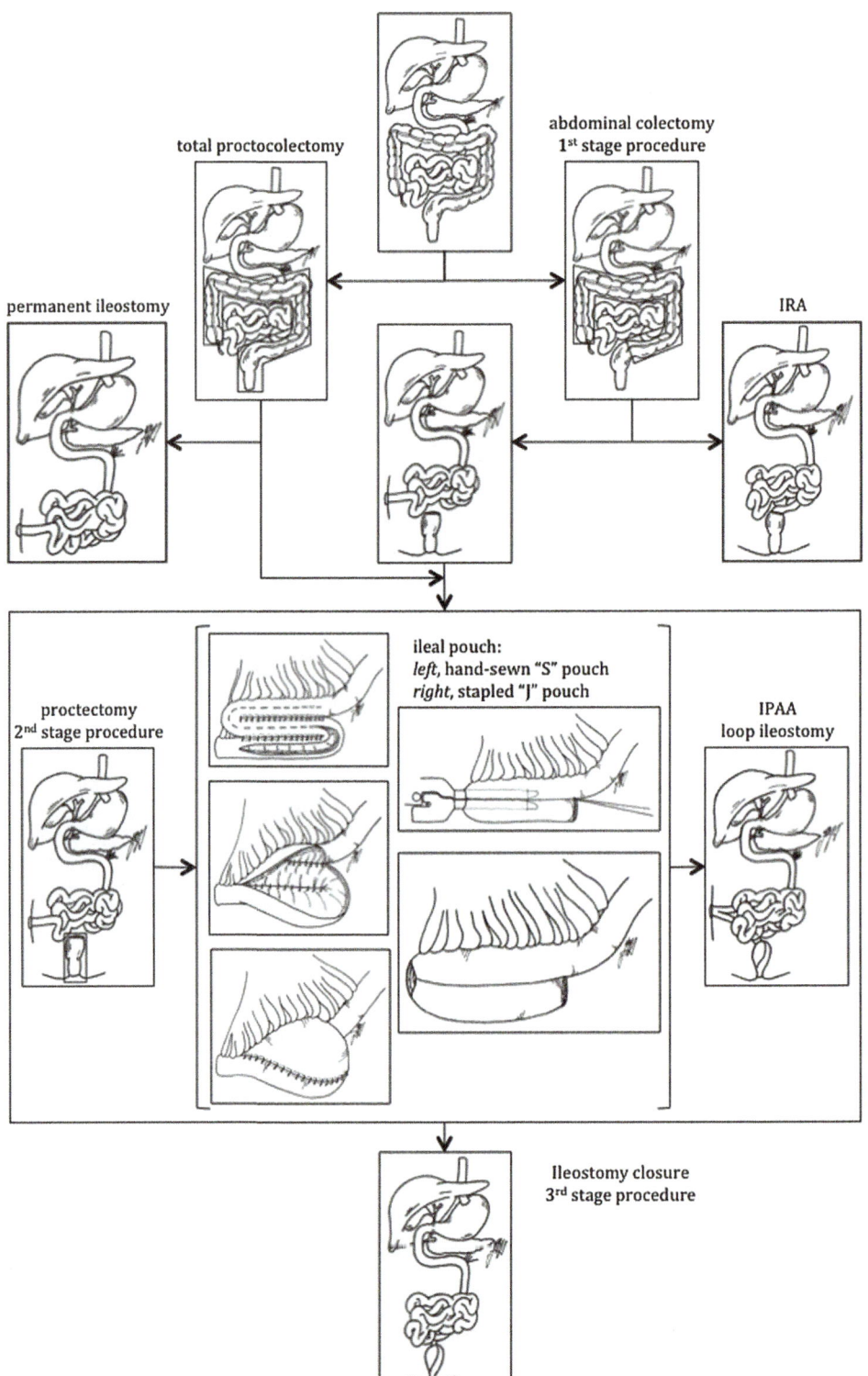

Fig. 14.3 Surgical decision-making algorithm

CRC. It is the procedure of choice for patients with impaired anal sphincter function, and distal or advanced rectal cancer. Other indications are the patient's choice of this procedure and the presence of systemic comorbidities contraindicating a restorative procedure. Total proctocolectomy with ileostomy has a low morbidity rate, it is a definitive procedure, but more than 50 % of the patients declare to have social and psychological problems due to the presence of the stoma [9, 13, 17]. In order to reduce patient's dissatisfaction with having a permanent stoma, Kock advocated the continent ileostomy in the 1970s [18]. In this procedure, the terminal ileum is intussuscepted within a pre-terminal ileal pouch forming a continent valve. Despite the theoretical advantages, the Kock's pouch is performed with decreasing frequency, due to high complications rate and failure of the continence mechanism in 40–50 % of the cases [19]. IRA for UC is not a common procedure. In fact, the rationale of this intervention is based on the presence of a minimal rectal involvement, quite a rare condition in UC. Nearly 60 % of the patients initially treated with IRA ultimately failed this procedure, requiring a completion proctectomy with or without a restorative IPAA [20]. In the past decades, a new role for IRA was advocated for fertile females in order to improve fecundity, which is at high risk after IPAA due to pelvic dissection and consequent adhesions [21]. However, results from tertiary IBD centres, that perform totally laparoscopic IPAA, have shown encouraging results in terms of fecundity and delivery, making laparoscopic IPAA the procedure of choice in young women [22].

Alan Parks and John Nicholls proposed the restorative proctocolectomy with IPAA in 1978, creating "an operation that permits total removal of all disease-prone mucosa in ulcerative colitis but avoids the need for a permanent ileostomy" [23]. IPAA is a very complex procedure, based on an extended colorectal resection and an autologous transplantation to create a new rectum using the small bowel, but it is also a "quality of life" surgery. After the nineties, well past the "learning curve", IPAA remains a highly demanding operation, with a low mortality rate in elective settings (0.2–1 %), but with a considerable morbidity. Early post-operative complication rates after IPAA vary between 28–58 %, and late complications in up to 52 %. Perioperative septic complications, related to the pouch and/or the ileo-anal anastomosis, are reported in the literature from 2.3–26.7 %. Long-term pouch failure rate ranges from 3 to 15 % [24–26]. Functional results and "quality of life" have been accessed by several studies, but with a wide variety of scores and methods and different follow-up. However, the evidence suggests that Health-Related Quality of Life (HRQoL) and Health Status (HS) of patients with ulcerative colitis improve 12 months after restorative proctocolectomy with IPAA, and are indistinguishable from the HRQoL and HS of the normal healthy population [27].

14.4 Surgical Techniques and Specific Complications

IPAA has become the preferred surgical option for the surgical treatment of UC. However, it remains a complex undertaking with the potential of remarkable short- and long-term morbidity. Successful outcomes are based upon careful patient selection, clear preoperative counselling, appropriate operative strategy and technique and adequate expertise of the surgical team in managing intraoperative problems and post-operative complications.

14.4.1 Staged Procedure

Restorative proctocolectomy may be performed as a 1-, 2- or 3-stage procedure (Fig. 14.3). A staged procedure is the procedure of choice in emergency, in acute severe colitis, when the patient is taking high dose of steroids (e.g. prednisolone >40 mg/day) or moderate steroid dose (20 mg/day) for more than 6 weeks, when differential diagnosis with CD is not established, when advanced CRC is present in the colon and in case of moderate to severe malnutrition [21].

Recent reports from Mayo Clinic and Cleveland Clinic have evidenced an increased risk of post-operative complications in patients undergoing restorative procedure under Infliximab therapy, suggesting a staged approach also for this setting [28, 29]. When appropriate skills are available, a laparoscopic approach is recommended [21]. A subtotal colectomy with end ileostomy, leaving in situ the rectum, is a relatively safe procedure even in critically ill patients, allowing patients to regain general health, normalize nutrition, interrupt any medical therapy (desaturating from steroids) and consider the option of an IPAA, an IRA or a permanent ileostomy [30, 31, 32]. There are specific recommendations on how to deal with the rectal stump, since these may have an impact on both complications and later proctectomy and IPAA. The whole rectum has to be preserved, with or without the distal part of the sigmoid colon, while dividing the rectum at the distal third is not recommended. In fact, pelvic dissection during the first procedure leads to high risk of nerves and sacral veins injury at the time of IPAA. Furthermore, post-operative pelvic fibrosis may impair ileo-anal anastomosis and jeopardize pouch function [21]. Blowout of the rectum in a very compromised bowel, due to a dehiscence of the closing suture, is the most common and dangerous complication of the staged procedure (Fig. 14.4). When necessary, a long rectal stump may allow performing a recto-cutaneous fistula, eliminating any sutured bowel from the abdominal cavity. Once again, the dehiscence of a too short rectal remnant in the pelvis should be impossible to be controlled and the consequent pelvic fibrotic reaction could lead to the impossibility of performing an IPAA.

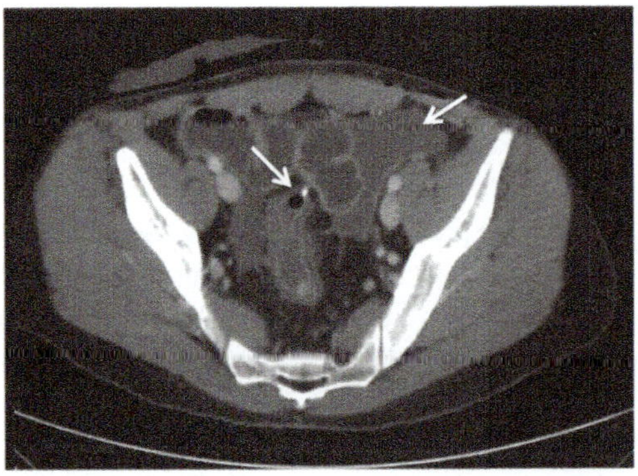

Proctectomy, pouch formation and ileo-anal anastomosis are the most technically demanding phases of the whole procedure. In elective cases, both resective (total proctocolectomy) and restorative (IPAA) procedures may be performed during the same intervention. Most surgeons favour creation of a temporary defunctioning loop ileostomy after IPAA to avoid anastomotic dehiscence and pelvic contamination; this is the classical two-stage procedure, since a second operation is needed, after 8–10 weeks, for ileostomy closure. However, some authors advocate the single stage procedure in selected cases, mainly on the basis of an exercise in risk management. Anastomotic dehiscence is three times higher in one-stage versus two-stage procedures (5 vs. 15 %), but ileostomy closure has the considerable complication rate of 11–25 %. So, the final decision is a balance between these two aspects, taking into account patient's specific risk factors (e.g. pre-operative therapy, nutrition, age, BMI, technical difficulties encountered during surgery) [33].

14.4.2 Pouch Configuration

Parks and Nicholls originally proposed a triple-limb S-shaped pouch, but several alternative designs have been described, including a high-capacity "W" pouch and an ease-to-perform "J" pouch [23, 34]. The evidence is that within 1 year after pouch construction, the pouch shape has no influence on functional results. However, different pouch designs have specific complications. The "S" pouch has an efferent limb that may suffer from kinking if it is longer than 1 cm, and a hand-sewn ileo-anal anastomosis with mucosectomy is necessary (see later). The "W" pouch avoids efferent limb complications, but is time-consuming with poor long-term benefits.

Fig. 14.4 32-year-old man in post-operative day 6 after laparoscopic total abdominal colectomy for acute colitis presenting with rectal stump dehiscence (*left arrow*) and visceral fluid collection (*right arrow*)

The "J" pouch is favoured by most surgeons because of the ease of construction, allows both manual or stapled anastomosis and less intestine is used in the process [35, 36].

14.4.3 Mucosectomy Versus Double Stapling

Dissection and removal of the columnar mucosa above the dentate line with trans-anal hand-sewn anastomosis was initially advocated in order to prevent UC recurrence and CRC. The main problem with mucosectomy is due to the removal of the anal transitional zone (ATZ), which is richly innervated by sensory nerve endings that mediate anal sampling reflexes, permitting discrimination of solids and liquids from gases and thus contributing to the whole continence mechanism (Fig. 14.5) [37]. Given that when performing an IPAA the maximum length of anorectal mucosa between the dentate line and the anastomosis should not exceed 2 cm (1–1.5 cm are better), a stapled IPAA is generally preferred since it improves continence through ATZ preservation and the cancer risk is equally low as in hand-sewn anastomosis (Figs. 14.6, 14.7) [21]. Even if the advent of reliable and ergonomic stapling instruments has

greatly simplified the pouch-anal anastomosis, the surgical team performing an IPAA has to be able to perform a hand-sewn anastomosis in case the stapler fails [21].

14.4.4 Laparoscopic IPAA

In referral centres a minimally invasive approach has become the standard of care. Avoidance of wound pain and complications, reduction of blood loss and adverse surgical events, improvements of short-term and long-term morbidity, reduction of adhesion formation preserving the risk of obstruction and fecundity and a better cosmesis in a young population, are all strong points of laparoscopic surgery [22, 38–41]. Laparoscopy, together with the application of enhanced recovery programmes, designed for early post-operative mobilization and feeding, is the new gold standard of care for UC patients.

14.4.5 Sexual Dysfunction, Fecundity, Pregnancy and Delivery

Rectal and pelvic dissection may result in damage of parasympathetic erigent nerves and sympathetic hypogastric plexus, regulating ejaculation in 1–4 % of the male patients. In

Fig. 14.5 Epithelial landmarks of the anorectal junction

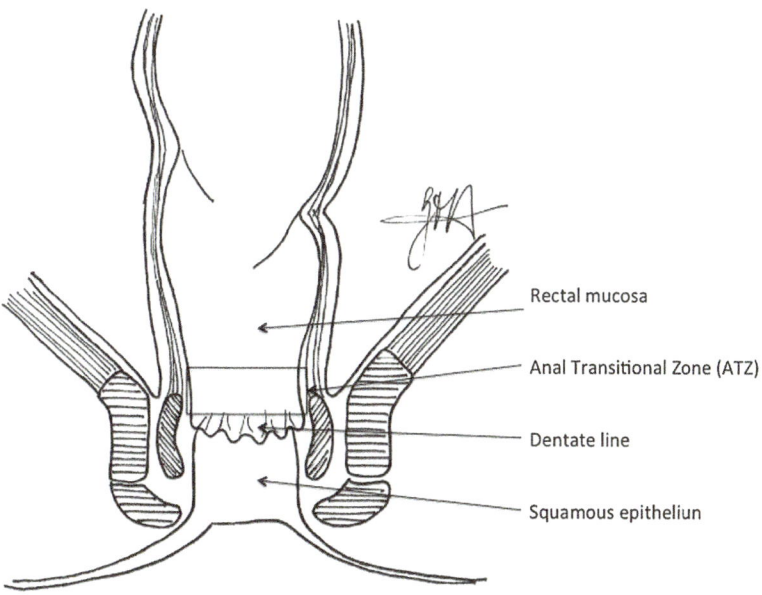

Rectal mucosa

Anal Transitional Zone (ATZ)

Dentate line

Squamous epitheliun

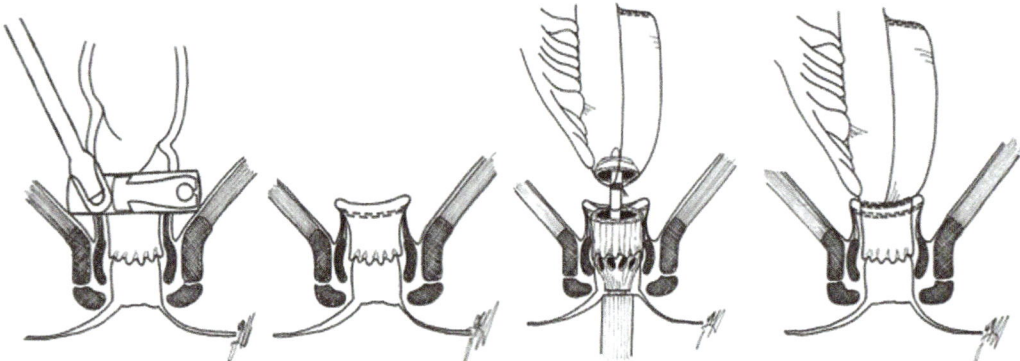

Fig. 14.6 Schematic representation of a stapled IPAA. Ultra-low rectal resection is performed by a gastro-intestinal-anastomosis (GIA) stapling device (*left*), while the IPAA is performed by a circular end-to-end anastomosis (CEEA) stapling device (*right*)

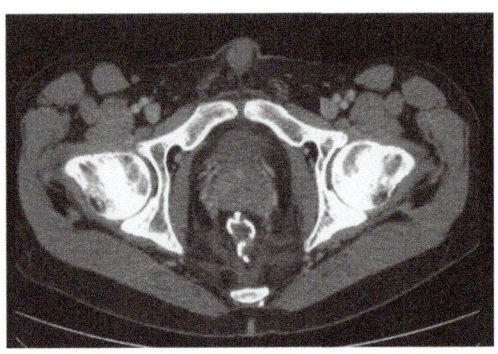

Fig. 14.7 Typical aspect of an ultra-low, stapled IPAA. The vertical limbs are the staple of the rectal resection performed by the GIA (they should be vertical or horizontal, depending on the intra-operative GIA positioning), while the circular are those of the IPAA performed by the CEEA

women, sexual dysfunction may be much higher at 8–11 %, mainly due to vaginal dryness, dyspareunia, pain interfering with sexual pleasure and limiting of sexual activity because of concerns of stool leakage [42]. However, impairment of sexual activity seems to improve in patients after IPAA compared to patients under intensive medical treatment (16 vs. 20 %), and 25 % of pouch patients refer better sex lives after surgery. In general, sexual dysfunction seems to be correlated to the global health status more than the restorative surgery [43].

Historically, pouch surgery was associated with a 98 % reduction in fertility, impaired by pelvic adhesions, but nowadays it may be preserved by laparoscopic surgery. As an alternative, abdominal colectomy with end ileostomy or IRA should be discussed with patients [21, 22].

During pregnancy, stool frequency and incontinence should worsen in the third trimester, due to the weight and dimensions of the uterus laying over the pouch, but pouch function quickly recovers to normal after delivery in 83 % of cases [44].

In the general population, delivery in primiparous and multiparous women is associated with a sphincter defect (often asymptomatic) on endosonography at 6 weeks, persisting at 6 months, of 35 and 44 %, respectively [45]. There is not enough evidence to recommend a particular mode of delivery in pouch women, but appropriate discussion with the patient is mandatory, since a major sphincter damage may lead to pouch failure and permanent ileostomy [21].

14.4.6 Pouch Failure and Salvage Surgery

In consideration of the high technical undertaking, the indication of performing the whole procedure by laparoscopy and the considerable early and late complications, IPAA should be performed only in specialist referral centres. Consistent evidence has been reported that patients undergoing surgery in high volume centres have reduced complication rates and better pouch salvage probability in the face of complications leading to pouch failure [21, 46, 47].

Pouch failure is defined as the need for pouch excision or indefinite defunctioning. There are four main causes for pouch failure: acute or chronic sepsis, poor function for mechanical or functional reasons, mucosal inflammation and neoplastic transformation [48]. Since IPAA surgery is an autologous transplantation and an anatomical reconstruction, but also a "quality of life" surgery, a careful clinical history and examination is essential to guide the clinician in discriminating pouch problem(s) and designing appropriate workup.

Endoscopy is very useful to obtain information on the mucosa status, such as cuffitis, pouchitis, Crohn's disease, dysplasia and cancer. Endoscopy, pouch enema and dynamic pouch defecography can be used for evaluation of pouch distensibility, afferent and efferent limb disorders and pouch prolapse or torsion. In most of the cases, a completion of the workup with a 2D/3D tomographic device is necessary. Computed Tomography (CT), Magnetic Resonance Imaging (MRI) and Ultrasonography (US) (either Endoanal or Transperineal) are very sensitive in identifying and characterizing septic problems and most mechanical disorders. In general, CT is preferred in emergency settings or in case a percutaneous drainage is needed, while MRI and US are used in elective condition in order to reduce X-ray exposure (Fig. 14.8).

In case of fistulas, abscesses, sinuses and IPAA stenosis, examination under anaesthesia (EUA) performed by an experienced surgeon is the crucial step for diagnosis and contemporary treatment of most conditions. In fact, the association of EUA with one of the tomographic imaging tools (CT, MRI, US) gives the best level of accuracy [49]. A large proportion of patients who experience post-operative pouch problems are successfully treated by transperineal approach, with or without faecal diversion. Dilation of IPAA stenosis is effective in 45–95 % of cases, but often multiple procedures are necessary. Both simple and complex septic

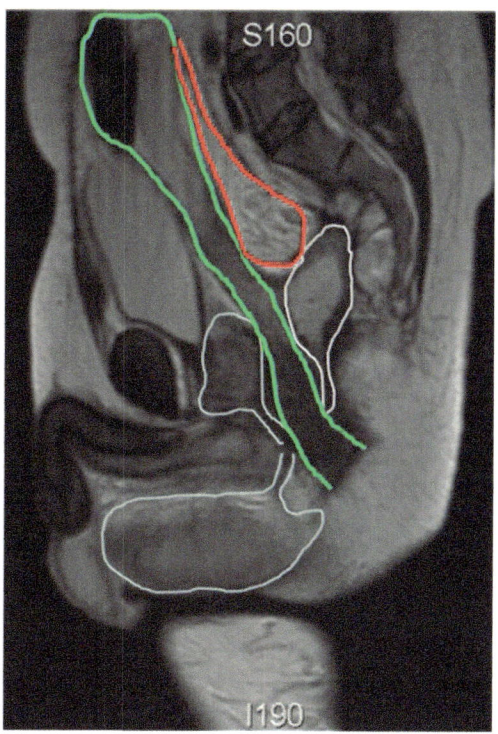

Fig. 14.8 MRI of a 46-year-old male patient presenting 13 months after restorative proctocolectomy and IPAA with multiple fistulae and abscesses. In *green* the pouch. In *red* the pouch mesentery. In *white* the perineal abscesses and fistulae

complications are manageable by EUA through abscess drainage, fistulotomy, fistulectomy, seton placement, sphincterotomy and mucosal advancement flaps. The more complex the septic complications, the higher is the risk of temporary stoma for prolonged periods [48, 50–52]. The most frequent mechanical causes of malfunctioning are a stenosis of IPAA, a too long efferent limb of an "S" pouch, a too long blind limb of a "J" pouch, a kinking of the afferent limb, twisting of the pouch, pouch intussusception, a too small pouch, megapouch and a too long rectal stump [53, 54].

Redo pouch is necessary when the IPAA has to be disconnected and the pouch revised or reconstructed through a combined transabdominal and transperineal approach. Obstructing problems should be managed using the existing pouch. For volume problems, specific procedures have been proposed in order to reduce or enlarge the pouch capacity. In case of septic complications the pouch itself is frequently involved, and thus a complete reconstruction is often necessary. Inflammatory disorders, due to a too long rectal stump or cuffitis, should be managed by complete removal of inflamed mucosa (completion of proctectomy and mucosectomy) and hand-sewn transanal anastomosis.

When performed by experienced surgeons in tertiary centres, redo pouch is a safe and effective procedure, with low mortality rate, complication rate from 19 to 51 %, success rate from 50 to 100 % and patients' quality of life satisfactory in 50–93 % of cases. Redo pouch surgery seems to have better results when performed for mechanical problems, instead of septic complications and when the original pouch is conserved, compared to pouch reconstruction [50–56].

14.4.7 Pouchitis

Pouchitis is a non-specific inflammation of the ileal reservoir and the most common complication of IPAA in patients with UC. Its frequency is related to the duration of follow-up, occurring in up to 50 % of patients 10 years after IPAA in large series from major referral centres. The cumulative incidence of pouchitis in patients with an IPAA for familial adenomatous polyposis is much lower, ranging from 0 to 10 %, for unknown reasons. Symptoms related to pouchitis include increased stool frequency and liquidity, abdominal cramping, urgency, tenesmus and pelvic discomfort, rectal bleeding and fever, even extraintestinal manifestations may occur. Pouchitis may present with sporadic acute episodes, but also with a chronic active indolent pattern. Endoscopy is mandatory for diagnosis, but MRI should be helpful in order to exclude concomitant complications such as mechanical or septic disorders and for the differential diagnosis with Crohn's disease. Depending on the characteristics of the pouch inflammation and possible complications, different therapeutic regimens are feasible, starting with antibiotics, through probiotics, up to immunomodulators and anti-TNF-α agents [1, 2, 15, 20, 21].

References

1. Ordas I, Eckmann L, Talamini M, Baumgart DC, Sandborn WJ (2012) Ulcerative colitis. Lancet 380:1606–1619
2. Danese S, Fiocchi C (2011) Ulcerative colitis. N Engl J Med 365:1713–1725
3. Gan SI, Beck PL (2003) A new look at toxic megacolon: an update and review of Incidence, etiology, pathogenesis, and management. Am J Gastroenterol 98:2363–2371
4. Fazio VW (1986) Toxic megacolon: natural history and management. In: Jagelman DG (ed) Mucosal ulcerative colitis. Futura, New-York, pp 159–161
5. Greensten AJ, Sachar DB, Gibas A, Schrag D, Heimann T, Janiwitz HD et al (1985) Outcome of toxic dilation in ulcerative and Crohn's colitis. J Clin Gastroenterol 7:137–139
6. Heppel J, Farkouh E, Dube S, Peloquin A, Morgan S, Bernard D (1986) Toxic megacolon, an analysis of 70 cases. Dis Colon rectum 29:789–792
7. Greenstein AJ, Barth JA, Sachar DB, Aufses AH Jr (1986) Free colonic perforation without dilatation in ulcerative colitis. Am J Surg 152:272–275
8. Michelassi F (1997) Indications for surgical treatment in ulcerative colitis and Crohn's disease. In: Michelassi F, Milson JW (eds) Operative strategies in inflammatory bowel disease. Springer, New-York, pp 150–153
9. Nicholls RJ (2002) Review article: ulcerative colitis—surgical indications and treatment. Aliment Pharmacol Ther 16:25–28
10. Wallaert JB, De Martino RR, Marsicovetere PS et al (2012) Venous thromboembolism after surgery for inflammatory bowel disease: are there modifiable risk factors? data from ACS NSQIP. Dis Colon Rectum 55:1138–1144
11. Cohen JL, Strong SA, Hyman NH (2005) Practice parameters for the surgical treatment of ulcerative colitis. Dis Colon Rectum 48:1997–2009
12. Berger M, Gribetz D, Korelitz BI (1975) Growth retardation in children with ulcerative colitis: the effect of medical and surgical therapy. Pediatrics 55:459–467
13. Hwang JM, Varma MG (2008) Surgery in inflammatory bowel disease. World J Gastroenterol 14:2678–2690
14. Eaden JA, Abrams KR, Mayberry JF (2001) The risk of colorectal cancer in ulcerative colitis: a meta-analysis. Gut 48:526–535
15. Van Assche G, Dignas A, Bokemeyer B et al (2013) Second European evidence-based consensus on the diagnosis and management of ulcerative colitis: special situations. J Crohns Colitis 7:1–33
16. Bernstein CN, Shanahan F, Weinstein WM (1994) Are we telling patients the truth about surveillance colonoscopy in ulcerative colitis? Lancet 343:71–74
17. Pemberton JH, Phillips SF, Dozois RR (1985) Current clinical results of conventional ileostomy.

In: Dozois RR (ed) Alternatives to conventional ileostomy. Year Book Medical Publisher, Chicago, p 40

18. Kock NG (1973) Continent ileostomy. Prog Surg 12:180

19. Dozois RR, Kelly KA, Bert RW, Beahrs OH (1980) Improved results with continent ileostomy. Ann Surg 192(3):319–324

20. Leijonmarck CE, Lofberg R, Ost A, Hellers G (1990) Long-term results of ileorectal anastomosis in ulcerative colitis in Stockholm County. Dis Colon Rectum 33:195–200

21. Dignass A, Lindsay JO, Sturm A et al (2012) Second European evidence-based consensus on the diagnosis and management of ulcerative colitis: current management. J Crohns Colitis. 6(10):991–1030

22. Bartels SA, D'Hoore A, Cuesta MA, Bensdorp AJ, Lucas C, Bemelman WA (2012) Significantly increased pregnancy rates after laparoscopic restorative proctocolectomy: a cross-sectional study. Ann Surg 256(6):1045–1048

23. Parks AG, Nicholls AJ (1978) Proctocolectomy without ileostomy for ulcerative colitis. Br Med J 2(6130):85–88

24. Fazio VW, Ziv Y, Church JM et al (1995) Ileal pouch-anal anastomosis: complications and function in 1005 patients. Ann Surg 222:120–127

25. Meagher AP, Farouk R, Dozois RR, Kelly KA, Pemberton JH (1998) J ileal pouch-anal anastomosis for chronic ulcerative colitis: complications and long-term outcome in 1310 patients. Br J Surg 85:800–803

26. Hueting WE, Buskens E, van der Tweel I, Gooszen HG, van Laarhoven CJHM (2005) Results and complications after pouch anal anastomosis: a meta-analysis of 43 observational studies comprising 9,317 patiens. Dig Surg 22:69–79

27. Heikens JT, de Vries J, van Laarhoven CJ (2012) Quality of life, health-related quality of life and health status in patients having restorative proctocolectomy with ileal pouch-anal anastomosis for ulcerative colitis: a systematic review. Colorectal Dis 14(5):536–544

28. Mor IJ, Vogel JD, da Luz Moreira A, Shen B, Hammel J, Remzi FH (2008) Infliximab in ulcerative colitis is associated with an increased risk of postoperative complications after restorative proctocolectomy. Dis Colon Rectum 51(8):1202–1207

29. Selvasekar CR, Cima RR, Larson DW et al (2007) Effect of infliximab on short-term complications in patients undergoing operation for chronic ulcerative colitis. J Am Coll Surg 204(5):956–962

30. Alves A, Panis Y, Bouhnik Y, Maylin V, Lavergne-Slove A, Valleur P (2003) Subtotal colectomy for severe acute colitis: a 20-year experience of a tertiary care center with an aggressive and early surgical policy. J Am Coll Surg 197:379–385

31. Berg DF, Bahadursingh AM, Kaminski DL, Longo WE (2002) Acute surgical emergencies in inflammatory bowel disease. Am J Surg 184:45–51

32. Hyman NH, Cataldo P, Osler T (2005) Urgent subtotal colectomy for severe inflammatory bowel disease. Dis Colon Rectum 48:70–73

33. Bach AP, Mortensen NJM (2006) Revolution and evolution: 30 years of ileoanal pouch surgery. Inflamm Bowel Dis 12:131–145

34. Utsunomiya J, Iwama T, Imajo M et al (1980) Total colectomy, mucosal proctectomy, and ileoanal anastomosis. Dis Colon Rectum 23:459–466

35. Johnston D, Williamson ME, Lewis WG et al (1996) Prospective controlled trial of duplicated (J) versus quadruplicated (W) pelvic ileal reservoirs in restorative proctocolectomy for ulcerative colitis. Gut 39:242–247

36. Oresland T, Fasth S, Nordgren S et al (1990) A prospective randomized comparison of two different pelvic pouch designs. Scand J Gastroenterol 25:986–996

37. Miller R, Bartolo DC, Orrom WJ et al (1990) Improvement of anal sensation with preservation of the anal transition zone after ileoanal anastomosis for ulcerative colitis. Dis Colon Rectum 33:414–418

38. Maartense S, Dunker MS, Slors JF et al (2004) Hand-assisted laparoscopic versus open restorative proctocolectomy with ileal pouch anal anastomosis: a randomized trial. Ann Surg 240:991–992

39. Antolovic D, Kienle P, Knaebel HP et al (2006) Totally laparoscopic versus conventional ileoanal pouch procedure-design of a single-centre, expertise based randomized controlled trial to compare the laparoscopic and conventional surgical approach in patients undergoing primary elective restorative proctocolectomy—LapConPouch-Trial. BMC Surg 6:13

40. Tilney HS, Lovegrove RE, Heriot AG, Purkayastha S, Constantinides V, Nicholls RJ, Tekkis PP (2007) Comparison of short-term outcomes of laparoscopic vs open approaches to ileal pouch surgery. Int J Colorectal Dis 22:531–542

41. El-Gazzaz GS, Kiran RP, Remzi FH, Hull TL, Geisler DP (2009) Outcomes of case-matched laparoscopically assisted versus open restorative proctocolectomy. Br J Surg 96:522–525

42. Bambrick M, Fazio VW, Hull TL, Pucel G (1996) Sexual function following restorative proctocolectomy in women. Dis Colon Rectum 39: 610–614

43. Farouk R, Pemberton JH, Wolff BG et al (2000) Functional outcomes after ileal pouch-anal anastomosis for chronic ulcerative colitis. Ann Surg 231:919–926

44. Ravid A, Richard CS, Spencer LM et al (2002) Pregnancy, delivery, and pouch function after ileal pouch-anal anastomosis for ulcerative colitis. Dis Colon Rectum 45:1283–1288

45. Sultan AH, Kamm MA, Hudson CN et al (1993) Anal-sphincter disruption during vaginal delivery. N Engl J Med 329:1905–1911

46. Burns EM, Bottle A, Aylin P et al (2011) Volume analysis of outcome following restorative proctocolectomy. Br J Surg 98:408–417

47. Raval MJ, Schnitzler M, O'Connor BI, Cohen Z, McLeod R (2007) Improved outcome due to increased experience and individualized management of leaks after ileal pouch-anal anastomosis. Ann Surg 246:763–770

48. Tulchinsky H, Cohen CRG, Nicholls RJ (2003) Salvage surgery after restorative proctocolectomy. Br J Surg 90:909–921

49. Van Assche G, Dignass A, Reinisch W, van der Woude CJ, Sturm A, De Vos M et al (2010) The second European evidence-based Consensus on the diagnosis and management of Crohn's disease: special situations. J Crohns Colitis 4(1):63–101

50. Sagar PM, Pemberton JH (2012) Intraoperative, postoperative and reoperative problems with ileoanal pouches. Br J Surg 99(4):454–468

51. Prudhomme M, Dozois RR, Godlewski G, Mathison S, Fabbro-Peray P (2003) Anal canal strictures after ileal pouch–anal anastomosis. Dis Colon Rectum 46:20–23

52. Zmora O, Efron JE, Nogueras JJ, Weiss EG, Wexner SD (2001) Reoperative abdominal and perineal surgery in ileoanal pouch patients. Dis Colon Rectum 44(9):1310–1314

53. Ehsan M, Isler JT, Kimmins MH, Billingham RP (2004) Prevalence and management of prolapse of the ileoanal pouch. Dis Colon Rectum 47(6):885–888

54. Maddireddy VK, Shorthouse A, Goodfellow P, Katory M (2007) Intermittent torsion of a megapouch: report of a case. Dis Colon Rectum 50(12):2244–2246

55. Shawki S, Belizon A, Person B, Weiss EG, Sands DR, Wexner SD (2009) What are the outcomes of reoperative restorative proctocolectomy and ileal pouch-anal anastomosis surgery? Dis Colon Rectum 52(5):884–890

56. Fazio VW, Wu JS, Lavery IC (1998) Repeat ileal pouch-anal anastomosis to salvage septic complications of pelvic pouches: clinical outcome and quality of life assessment. Ann Surg 228(4):588–597

Imaging of Ileal Pouch Surgery and Related Complications

15

Massimo Tonolini

Over the last few decades, surgical treatment of ulcerative colitis (UC) has been refined to offer patients needing colectomy a better quality of life. Initially described 30 years ago, restorative proctocolectomy (RPC) with ileal pouch-anal anastomosis (IPAA) has become the "gold standard" surgical procedure. Its rationale includes complete removal of the diseased bowel with reduction of lifetime cancer risk, combined with preservation of anal sphincter function allowing patients an unchanged body image without ileostomy, and an acceptable lifestyle with preserved anal defecation route [1–4].

As discussed elsewhere in this volume, according to the European Crohn's and Colitis Organization (ECCO) guidelines, the main indications for RPC include severe colitis refractory to medical treatment, patients who remain steroid-dependent for more than 6 weeks, and detection of dysplastic changes or carcinoma. In the 1990s, colectomy rates after 10 years with UC approached 23–34 %, and reached 35–54 % with extensive disease. Currently, 10-year colectomy rates are 18 % for extensive UC at diagnosis, as low as 2 % for proctitis and distal disease and 39 % for the few patients with proctitis who subsequently progress to extensive UC [2, 3].

A staged procedure including subtotal colectomy, ileal pouch creation and temporary covering loop ileostomy as the first step is usually considered a wise surgical choice, since it allows to cure the burden of colitis, and to regain nutritional status and general health. Before recanalization surgery, the patient has time to consider the lifelong option of an IPAA. Alternatively, a one-stage surgical treatment without ileostomy is increasingly performed [2, 3].

However, despite general patient satisfaction with the preserved faecal continence, RPC with IPAA is associated with a significant long-term morbidity approaching 70 % after 10 years, and with a non-negligible (4–15 %) rate of pouch failure leading to excision and permanent ileostomy. The very low perioperative mortality is mostly related to the young age of many patients [5–7].

Evidence exists that patients operated in specialized institutions performing a large number of procedures have better outcomes than those operated in limited-volume centers. Therefore, it is advisable that RPC-IPAA surgery should be performed by experienced surgeons [2, 3].

Recently, a classification of ileal pouch-related disorders has been proposed by Shen, Fazio et al. which distinguishes surgical and mechanical complications from inflammatory and infectious conditions, functional disorders, dysplasia/neoplasia and metabolic systemic changes. Surgical and mechanical complications include anastomotic leaks, pelvic sepsis and abscesses, pouch sinuses and fistulas, strictures, afferent or

M. Tonolini (✉)
Radiology Department, "Luigi Sacco" University Hospital, Via G.B. Grassi 74, 20157 Milan, Italy
e-mail: mtonolini@sirm.org

M. Tonolini (ed.), *Imaging of Ulcerative Colitis*,
DOI: 10.1007/978-88-470-5409-7_15, © Springer-Verlag Italia 2014

efferent limb syndromes, portal vein thrombi, sexual dysfunction and infertility. Inflammatory abnormalities include pouchitis, which is the commonest long-term IPAA complication, along with cuffitis, Crohn's disease (CD) of the pouch, proximal small-bowel overgrowth and inflammatory polyps. Irritable pouch syndrome and anismus are categorized as functional pouch disorders, whereas anemia and osteopenia are the usual metabolic complications [7].

In the majority of cases, pouch failure requiring permanent ileostomy is due to persistent dysfunction, septic complications, a missed diagnosis of CD and rarely to refractory pouchitis. Best performed in specialized institutions, salvage surgery may reach a 50 % success rate with acceptable functional outcomes [2, 3].

15.1   Imaging Techniques and Normal Pouch Anatomy

In the past, fluoroscopic pouchography using water-soluble iodinated contrast (Gastrografin, Bracco, or Gastromiro, Bayer-Schering) administered through the temporary ileostomy, or retrogradely through the anus, was routinely performed to image possible IPAA-related complications. Radiographic pouchography allowed distension and anatomic definition of the pouch reservoir, created by folding the terminal ileum on itself with side-to-side anastomosis. Furthermore, although without cross-sectional information about the surrounding planes, fluoroscopic studies enabled opacification of anastomotic leaks and fistulas and detection of strictures [8–10].

Currently, standard supine and upright abdominal radiographs are initially requested in most cases when patients with history of IPAA surgery present to the emergency department with acute abdominal symptoms. Plain films allow to detect intraperitoneal free air consistent with perforation, bowel gas distension and air-fluid levels suggesting obstruction. However, radiographs provide extremely limited information about pouch abnormalities.

More recently, computed tomography (CT) has been adopted to diagnose IPAA-related septic complications, allowing assessment of both pouch and surrounding structures. Currently, multidetector CT (MDCT) is universally available, extremely fast in acquisition and increasingly performed to investigate patients with IPAA, particularly when early complications are suspected during post-operative hospitalization. Unless contraindicated by allergy or impaired renal function, intravenous injection of iodinated contrast medium is routinely used. In most cases, a single contrast-enhanced MDCT acquisition during the portal venous phase is sufficient, whereas multiple acquisitions should be discouraged to avoid additional radiation dose. Peroral or rectal bowel opacification with water-soluble iodinated contrast may be useful when leakage is suspected, or for problem solving [9–11].

When interpreting MDCT studies, image review should routinely include sagittal and coronal reformations that are highly helpful to clarify the post-operative anatomy. The normal ileal pouch appears as a fluid-filled structure with the presence of metallic staples opposed 180° to each other. The pouch-anal anastomosis, if performed with mechanical devices, may be also identifiable by the presence of hyperattenuating clips (Fig. 15.1) [8–11].

In selected patients with chronic obstructive symptoms, an MDCT-enterography technique including small bowel distension via peroral ingestion of hyperdense or neutral enteral contrast material (such as polyethylene-glycol solution) may be beneficial to investigate low-grade or intermittent intestinal obstructive states [12–14].

More recently, pelvic magnetic resonance imaging (MRI) is increasingly used for the assessment of pouch-related inflammatory conditions. MRI provides an accurate multiplanar assessment of normal IPAA post-operative anatomy, and identification of possible complications. As from previous experiences with perianal inflammatory disease, intrinsic MRI advantages include its multiplanar capability, panoramic and detailed view, superb contrast resolution and possibility to suppress fat

Fig. 15.1 Normal MDCT imaging appearance of an endoscopically unremarkable ileal pouch as seen on sagittal (**a**), coronal (**b**) and axial (**c**) images. Well distended by fluid-faecal content (*), the pouch reservoir occupies the original anatomic site of the rectum, and is identified by the presence of metallic staples facing each other (*arrows*). More caudally (**d**), the pouch-anal anastomosis is also identifiable (*arrowhead*) [Partly reprinted with permission from Ref. [11]]

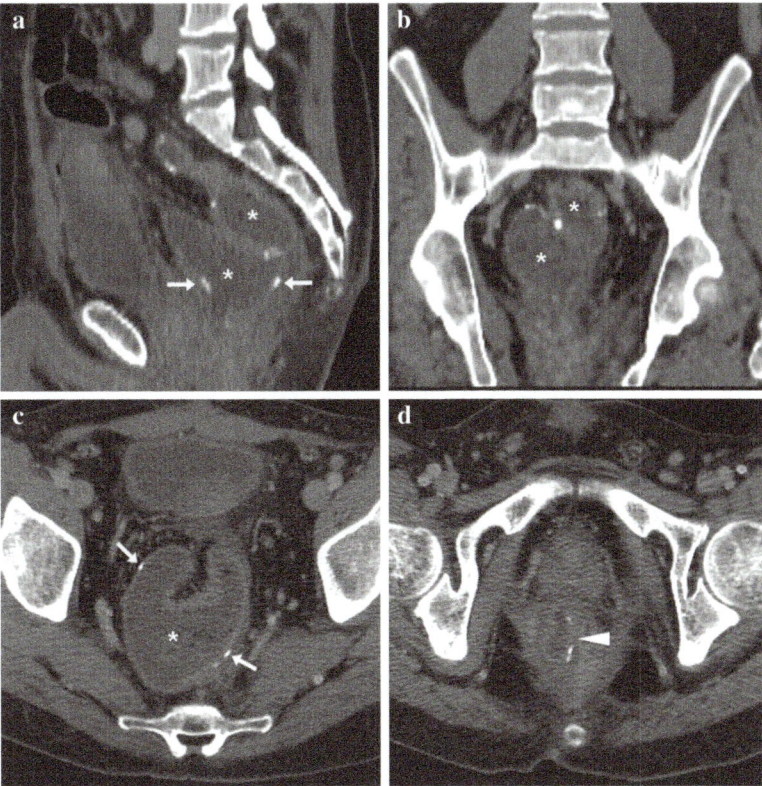

background, excellent visualization of abscesses and fistulas even with closed orifices, and detection of enhancement corresponding to inflammatory activity [10, 11, 15–17].

MRI is feasible even in patients with anal stenosis or pain, and its lack of irradiation and limited biologic invasiveness of gadolinium contrast are particularly beneficial in young patients who may need repeated imaging. MRI is performed with a phased-array coil positioned on the pelvis without any special patient preparation. Our protocol includes precontrast acquisition of multiplanar T2-weighted sequences, axial T1-weighted and fat-saturated (STIR) images. After intravenous paramagnetic contrast administration, enhanced multiplanar T1-weighted sequences are acquired, with fat suppression in at least one plane. Additionally, thin-section images may be planned on the perianal and perineal region if clinical or imaging findings suggest its possible involvement [11].

Similarly to MDCT, the ileal pouch is identified at MRI from the small ferromagnetic artefacts with signal voids on all sequences, due to the metallic staples (Fig. 15.2) [11, 15, 16].

The best accuracy in diagnosing complex IPAA-related disorders is achieved by a combination of pouch endoscopy with at least one imaging modality such as water-soluble contrast enema, MDCT and MRI [18]. According to our personal experience, pelvic MRI is highly valuable to complement pouch endoscopy in patients with proven or suspected pouchitis, abscesses or fistulas, to allow the differentiation of simple pouchitis from pelvic sepsis, which has been found even in patients with normal endoscopic findings and usually requires an aggressive therapy. Alternatively, when obstruction is suspected, contrast enema or MDCT may be performed before or after endoscopy to provide a more panoramic view of the entire abdomen and pelvis [11, 18].

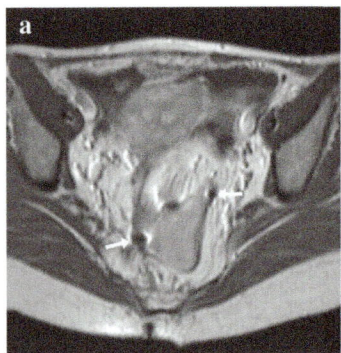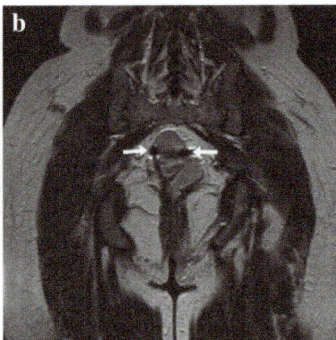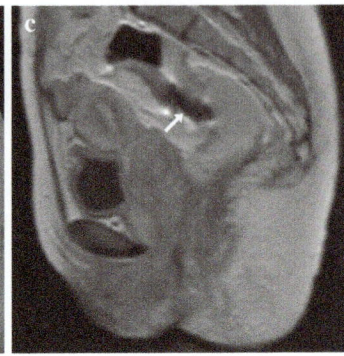

Fig. 15.2 Usual MRI appearance of a normal, moderately distended ileal pouch on axial T1- (**a**), coronal T2- (**b**) and post-contrast sagittal T1-weighted (**c**) images, with small ferromagnetic artefacts opposed to each other and due to presence of metallic staples (*arrows*) [Partly reprinted with permission from Ref. [11]]

15.2 Surgical and Mechanical Post-operative Complications

In our experience, cross-sectional imaging is often requested during the post-operative hospitalization following RPC−IPAA procedures when early surgical complications are suspected. In the majority of patients, indication for urgent studies include persistent abdominal pain, tenderness or peritonitis, fever, abnormal drainage from tubes, failure to achieve canalization and laboratory signs indicating blood loss or elevated acute phase reactants.

Although plain abdominal radiographs sometimes provide useful information, in most instances prompt investigation with contrast-enhanced MDCT is beneficial for comprehensive assessment of the abdomen and pelvis, and is felt highly helpful by our surgeons to guide the patient's management.

When performing and interpreting imaging studies in patients with recent or previous IPAA surgery, precise knowledge of surgical technique details and timing is needed to elucidate early post-operative conditions that may sometimes require reintervention. On the basis of our experience, we recommend a consistent approach to study interpretation, whether it refers to problems occurring after the first surgical procedure (subtotal colectomy, ileal pouch creation and covering loop ileostomy), following

ileostomy takedown, or after a one-stage procedure without temporary ileostomy. The different elements characteristic of RPC-IPAA surgery should be thoroughly reviewed, including the ileal pouch–anal anastomosis, the morphology and distension of the pouch reservoir including its afferent and efferent limbs, the peripouch fat planes and the ileostomy (Fig. 15.3).

15.2.1 Anastomotic Dehiscence and Leaks

Defined by Shen, Fazio et al. as "anastomotic separation leading to exodus of pouch luminal content", anastomotic leak most usually occurs at the pouch-anal anastomosis, whereas less common sites include the tip of the J pouch, and the pouch body along the staple line [7].

Although small leaks may not cause pelvic sepsis, anastomotic dehiscence is a critical diagnosis that usually dictates surgical reintervention and repair, and requires prolonged faecal diversion, suture lines should be carefully scrutinized on MDCT. In the past, contrast extravasation during pouchography in the soft tissues surrounding the pouch-anal anastomosis was the diagnostic hallmark of leakage [8–10].

Currently, MDCT represents the first-line investigation in most instances. Although the anastomotic leak may not be directly identified, MDCT is extremely sensitive for the detection of

Fig. 15.3 Approach to interpretation of an early post-operative MDCT study. Multiplanar examination review should focus on the pouch-anal anastomosis (*arrowhead* in **a**), morphology and size of the pouch reservoir (*) including its afferent and efferent limbs (**b**) and sutures (**c**), the peripouch fat planes and the presence and features of the ileostomy (**c, d**)

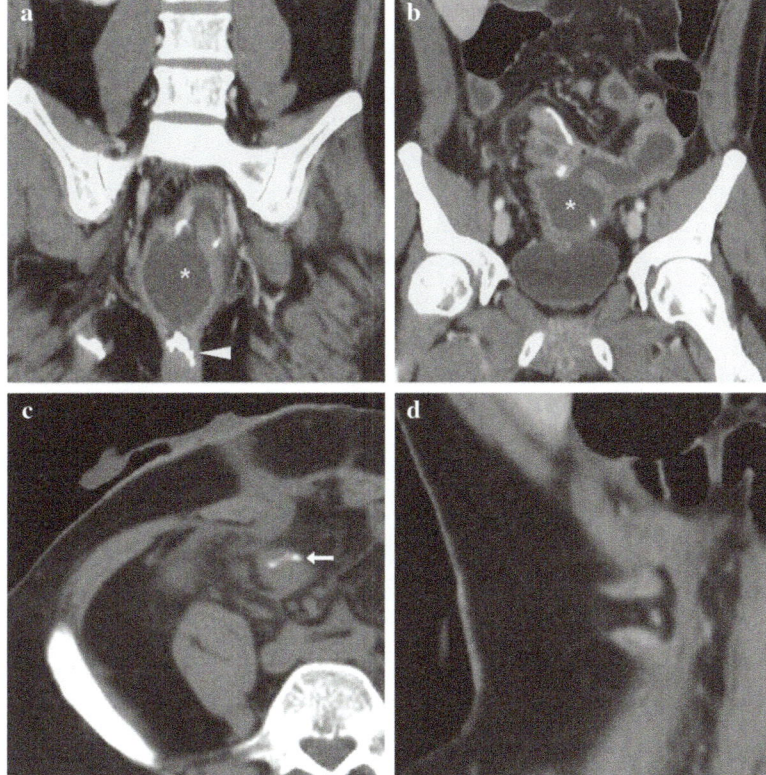

extraluminal air (Fig. 15.4a, b), fluid collections or hyperattenuating contrast material (Fig. 15.4c, d). These findings should be sought for, and reported as abnormal, since they strongly suggest anastomotic dehiscence [8–10, 15, 16].

Finally, persistent intraperitoneal air and MDCT findings suggesting peritonitis (Fig. 15.5) should alert the possible presence of extraluminal leak, even with normal appearances at the ileostomy and surgical anastomoses.

15.2.2 Post-operative Pelvic Sepsis, Pouch Abscesses, Sinuses and Fistulas

The definition of IPAA-related pelvic sepsis includes any infectious process developing in the peripouch area or distally to the pelvic inlet. Clinical manifestations may include local pain, purulent discharge from fistulous orifices, fever

and abnormal acute phase reactants, sometimes vaginal drainage, pneumaturia, fecaluria or frequent urinary tract infections [7]. Globally, pelvic sepsis is diagnosed with a prevalence of 6–37 %, and represents the main cause of pouch failure in UC patients, leading to pouch excision of 30 % of cases, and is associated with a 3 % mortality rate [5–7].

Early post-operative sepsis occurs in 5–20 % of patients undergoing RPC with IPAA. Even in the absence of demonstrable anastomotic leaks, on post-operative MDCT studies abnormal collections suggesting pelvic sepsis should be carefully sought for, particularly nearby the ileostomy site and surgical anastomoses. The MDCT hallmark of an abscess is represented by a fluid-like collection surrounded by a well-defined, variable-thickness enhancing rim (Fig. 15.6a, b). Alternative diagnoses such as fluid-attenuating serous (Fig. 15.6c) or hyperattenuating hemorrhagic collections (Fig. 15.6d)

Fig. 15.4 Early
dehiscence of the ileal
pouch–anal anastomosis
identified on axial (**a**) and
coronal (**b**) MDCT images
by extraluminal air leak on
the *right* side (*arrowheads*)
that required surgical
reoperation. In a different
patient, MDCT acquisition
after peroral administration
of hyperattenuating iodine-
based contrast medium (**c**,
d) reveals extraluminal
collection (*) opacified
through a contrast leak
(*arrowhead* in **c**), a finding
that prompted surgical
reintervention with pouch
excision and permanent
ileostomy

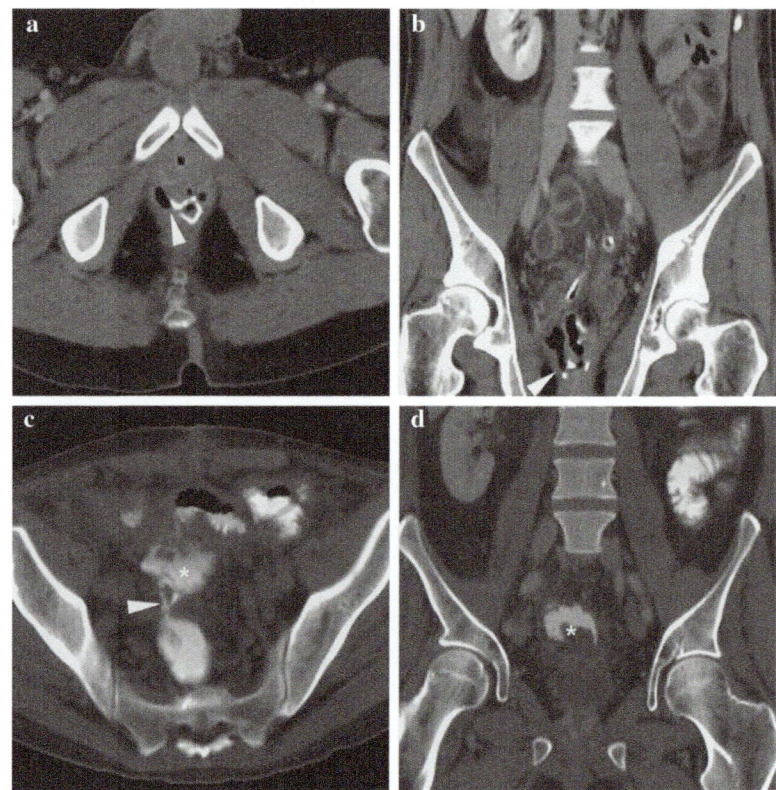

may be proposed on the basis of imaging findings [15, 16].

In the majority of cases, early post-operative
sepsis results from leakage at the site of the
pouch-anal anastomosis (Fig. 15.7). Whereas a
sinus is a blind tract that originates from the
pouch-anal anastomosis (Fig. 15.8) and may
lead to the formation of an abscess, a pouch-
related fistula involves an abnormal communi-
cation between any level of the ileal pouch
epithelium and a different structure, such as the
ischioanal space, perineal skin and subcutaneous
planes, vagina or urinary bladder (Fig. 15.9).
Both entities usually result from a later presentation of an initial anastomotic leak [7, 11].

MDCT promptly reveals abnormal peripouch
collections, but is rather insensitive for the
presence of leaks, sinuses (Fig. 15.8) and fistulas. Conversely, due to its soft-tissue contrast
MRI exquisitely identifies oedematous tissue,

fluid structures and inflammatory contrast
enhancement suggesting acute inflammation.
Usually located posteriorly to the pouch reservoir, abscesses are seen as fluid collections that
tend to layer dependently, may contain gas
pockets and have mass effect (Figs. 15.7, 15.8,
15.10). The underlying presence of a sinus tract
giving rise to a peripouch abscess may be
demonstrated directly as extraluminal leak of
retrogradely injected contrast during pouchography (Fig. 15.8), or identified on MRI images
as a fluid-filled hyperintense tubular track of
variable length (Fig. 15.7). On post-contrast
acquisitions, inflamed granulation tissue in the
walls of abscesses, sinuses and fistulas enhances,
whereas fluid in tracts and purulent abscess
content remain T1-hypointense (Figs. 15.7,
15.8, 15.10). Perianal and pouch-vaginal fistulas
are discussed in depth in Chap. 13 of this book
[11, 15, 16].

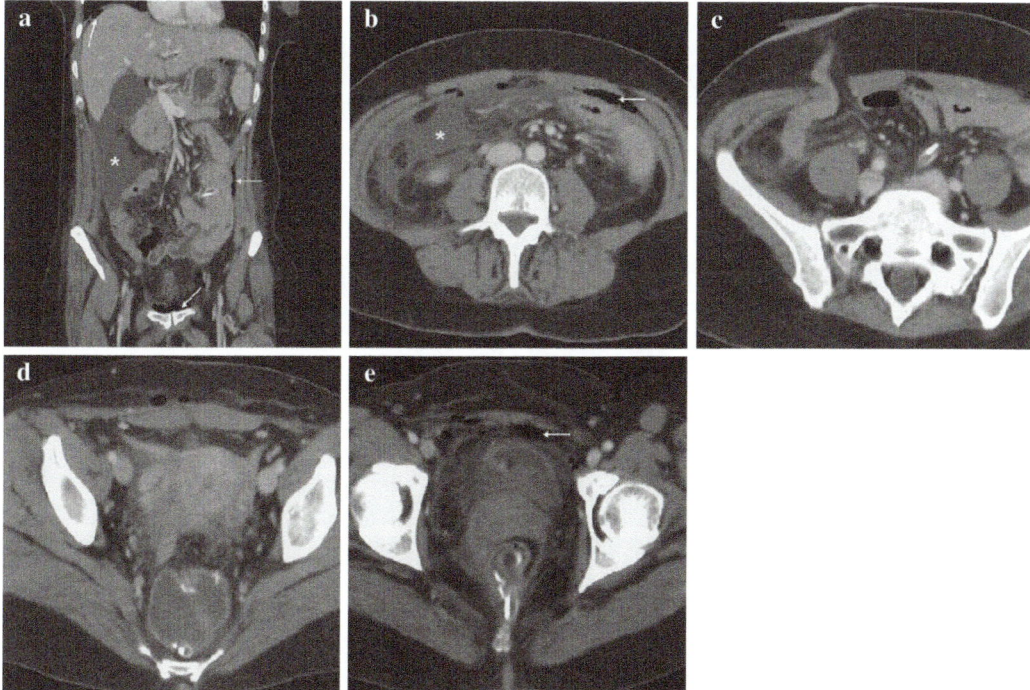

Fig. 15.5 Peritonitis following proctocolectomy with J pouch creation and ileostomy. Multiplanar MDCT images show peritoneal fluid (*) and serosal thickening, persistent air in the peritoneal cavity and subperitoneal Retzius' space (thin *arrows*), and normal appearances of the ileostomy (**c**), ileal pouch (**d**) and pouch-anal anastomosis (**e**). Reintervention confirmed biliary peritonitis due to focal ileal rupture above the ileostomy that was repaired

15.2.3 Bowel Obstruction and Strictures

Following RPC–IPAA surgery, strictures are a common occurrence (9.2 % of patients) with both stapled and hand-sewn anastomosis, that are categorized according to their site, as anastomotic or pouch outlet, midpouch, pouch inlet and afferent limb strictures. Strictures may be inflammatory or fibrotic in nature, and result from either inappropriate surgical technique, ischaemia, or concurrent use of nonsteroidal anti-inflammatory drugs [5, 7].

In patients with obstructive symptoms such as abdominal distension and pain, nausea or vomiting, plain radiographs are helpful as a first-line investigation to confirm clinical suspicion and estimate the degree of obstruction. Cross-sectional imaging provides precise assessment of the presence, level and severity of obstruction, thereby allowing a correct therapeutic choice and planning of endoscopic or bougie dilatation, stricturoplasty, pouch diversion or excision [7, 19, 20].

During the early post-operative period, small-bowel obstruction occurs in nearly one-third of patients, resulting from adhesions, strictures or volvulus. At MDCT, the hallmark of obstruction includes a focal bowel wall thickening (most often along a staple line), upstream dilatation with abundant endoluminal fluid, air-fluid levels and occasionally the small bowel faeces sign (Fig. 15.11a, b). In our experience, post-operative obstruction frequently occurs at the site of the closed previous ileostomy, at the inner surface of the anterior abdominal wall (Fig. 15.11c, d) [8, 9, 15].

In patients with history of RPC-IPAA surgery and low-grade or intermittent obstruction, MDCT enterography is indicated to investigate the site and probable cause of symptoms.

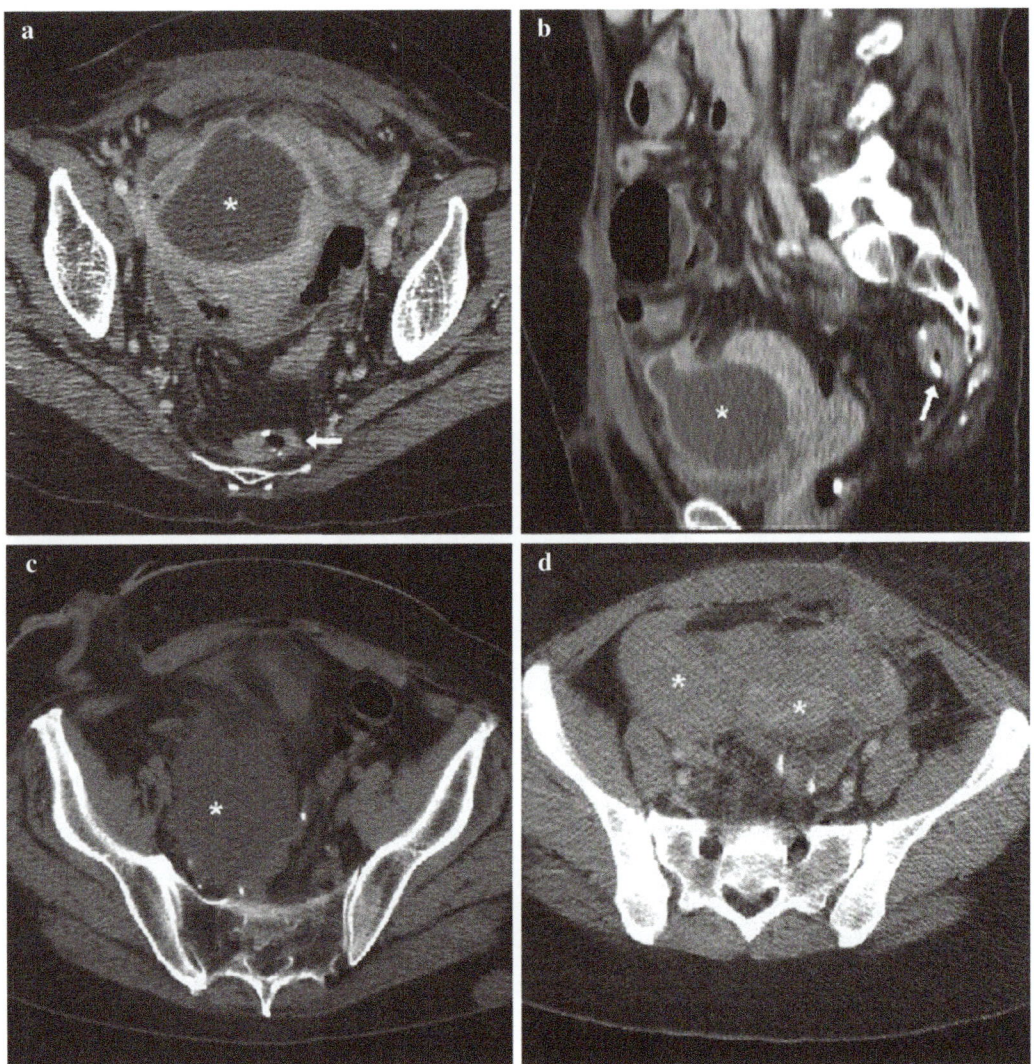

Fig. 15.6 Pelvic abscess collection (**a**, **b**) with enhancing rim and internal fluid-like content following proctocolectomy. Note normal appearance of the collapsed ileal pouch (*arrows*). In another patient with ileostomy (**c**), a fluid-attenuating collection without perceptible walls (*) corresponded to serous fluid at evacuation. In a third patient (**d**), extensive hyperattenuating haemorrhage (*) was detected in the Retzius' subperitoneal space

Stricture often occurs at the pouch inlet and site of ileal–pouch recanalization following ileostomy takedown, which is usually found in the right iliac fossa (Figs. 15.12, 15.13) [15].

Stenosis of the pouch-anal anastomosis is diagnosed at clinical examination in approximately 8–14 % of patients, although with greatly variable obstructive symptoms, and is usually treated effectively by means of dilatation under anaesthesia. Anal stenosis is suggested on cross-sectional imaging as mural thickening of the affected perianastomotic area associated with upstream bowel overdistension with fluid, stool or both, and can be confirmed by means of contrast fluoroscopy (Figs. 15.13, 15.14) [5, 10, 11, 21, 22].

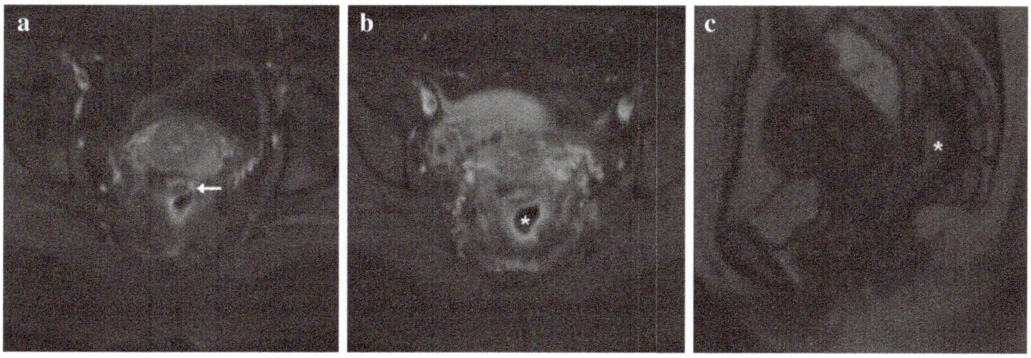

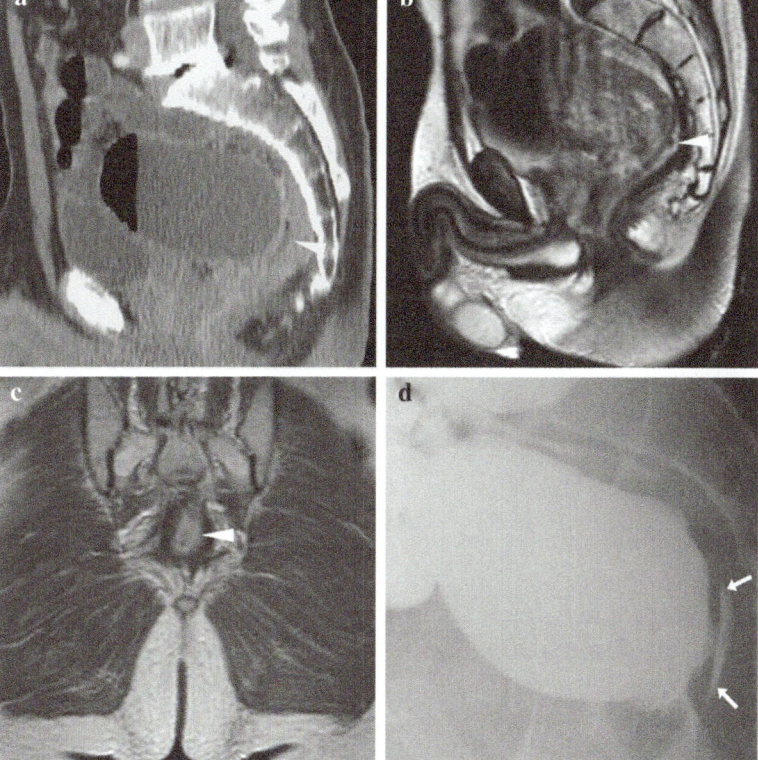

Fig. 15.7 Pelvic sepsis in a patient with perineal pain and purulent discharge. MRI shows dehiscence at the pouch-anal anastomosis as an enhancing leak (*arrow* in **a**) giving rise to a large retropouch abscess (*) [Reprinted with permission from Ref. [11]]

Fig. 15.8 Pouch sinus in a patient with chronic low-grade pelvic sepsis, endoscopic detection of fistulous orifices at the pouch-anal anastomosis. Contrast-enhanced MDCT (**a**) and MRI (**b, c**) detect an enhancing structure with central fluid-like structure (*arrowheads*) located behind the dilated ileal pouch reservoir. Fluoroscopic pouchography (**d**) detects contrast extravasation (*arrows*) opacifying the central portion, indicating the presence of a pouch sinus

15.2.4 Portal Venous System Thrombosis

As more extensively discussed in Chap. 9 of this book, thrombosis of the portal venous system is frequently (in 39–45 % of cases) detected on MDCT performed after RPC-IPAA surgery [23].

Therefore, when interpreting early post-operative imaging studies the splenic, mesenteric, portal and intrahepatic veins should be carefully scrutinized for filling defects. In most cases venous thrombi are multiple, peripheral and occlusive, whereas central thrombi in the main veins tend to be non-occlusive [7, 23–25].

Fig. 15.9 Pouch-vesical
fistula clinically diagnosed
by onset of fecaluria.
Coronal (**a**) and sagittal
(**b**) CT reformations depict
fistulization (*arrows*) of
pouch limb to the bladder
dome [Reprinted with
permission from Ref. [11]]

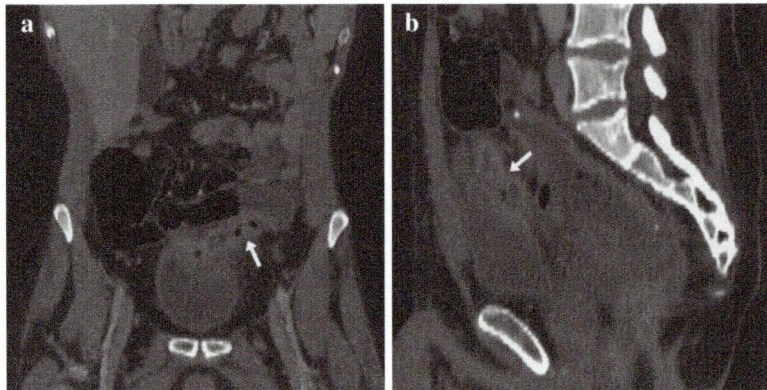

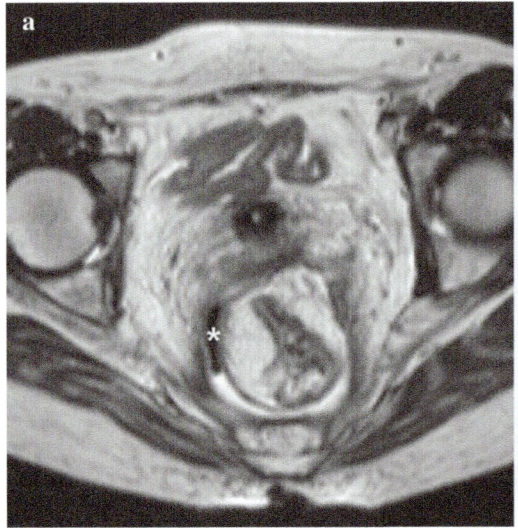
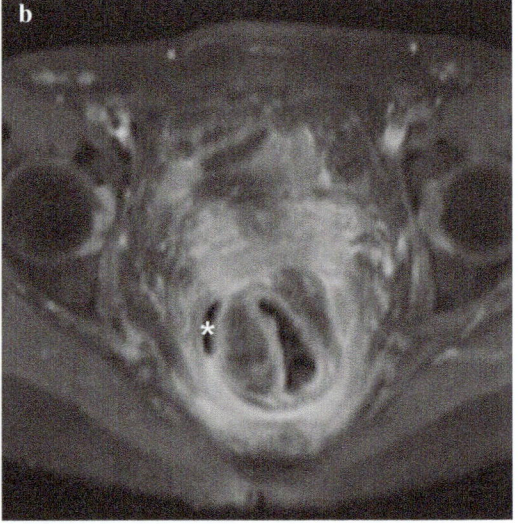

Fig. 15.10 Chronic sepsis with fever and pelvic dis-comfort. Axial T2 (**a**) and post-contrast fat-suppressed T1-weighted (**b**) images document a large horseshoe-shaped abscess collection (*) with a gas-fluid level in the site of the mesorectal fascia [Partly reprinted with permission from Ref. [11]]

15.3 Inflammatory Conditions

By far the most common pouch-related compli-cation, pouchitis is a non-specific inflammation of the ileal reservoir that may be recurrent or persistent. Its pathophysiology is poorly under-stood, and probably involves an abnormal immune response to altered bacterial flora, lead-ing to acute and/or chronic inflammation [1, 4, 7].

Exceedingly rare in patients operated with an IPAA for familial adenomatous polyposis, pouchitis is very common in UC patients.

Reported risk factors include extensive UC dis-ease, associated extraintestinal manifestations (particularly primary sclerosing cholangitis), being a non-smoker, p-ANCA positive serology and regular use of nonsteroidal anti-inflamma-tory drugs [1, 4]. The incidence of pouchitis related to the duration of the follow-up, and its cumulative risk is estimated in the range 23–46 % at 10 years after IPAA in large series from major referral centres [5, 7, 21, 26, 27].

Pouchitis is diagnosed clinically, on the basis of characteristic symptoms such as increased stool frequency and fluidity, urgency or

Fig. 15.11 Small bowel obstruction following one-stage RPC with IPAA. Coronal (**a**) and axial (**b**) MDCT images show "beaking" of the ileum at the site of a surgical clip, with upstream dilatation, endoluminal fluid and air-attenuation feces. During reintervention, obstruction was confirmed and treated with adhesiolysis, and resection of an 80-cm-long ileal segment. In a different patient, shortly after recanalization procedure MDCT (**c**, **d**) shows stricture at the previous ileostomy site, causing upstream bowel dilatation

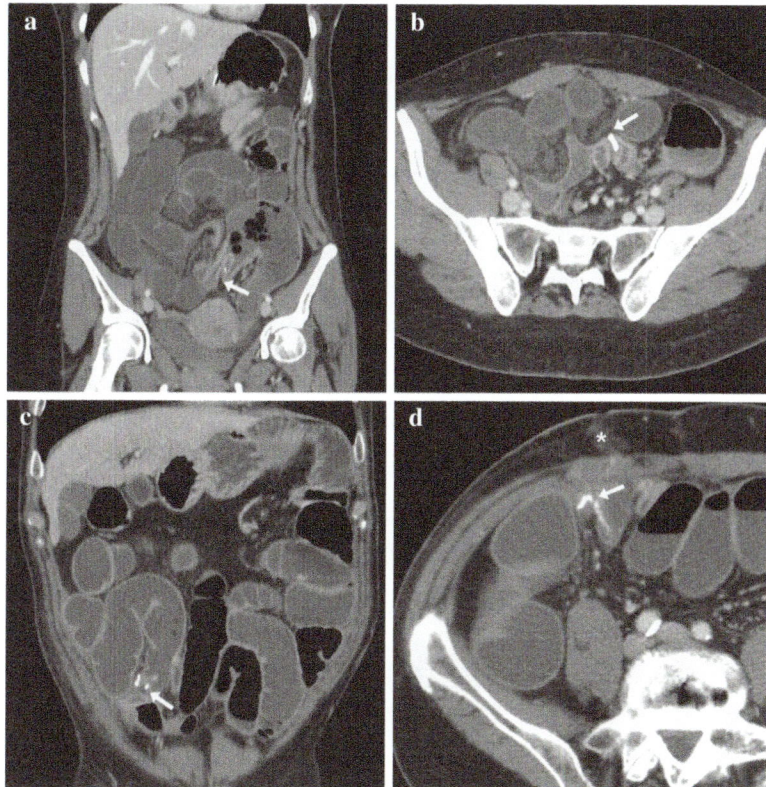

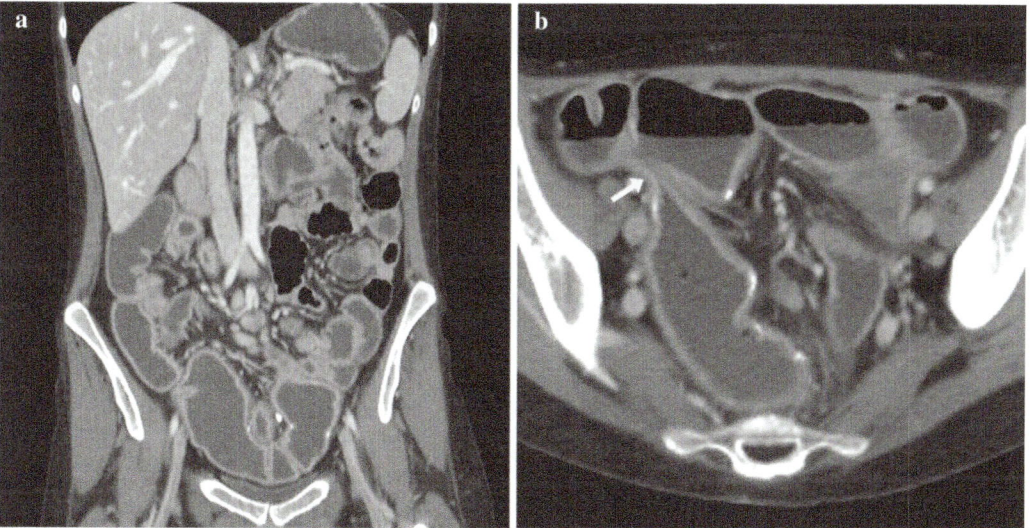

Fig. 15.12 Intermittent obstruction in a patient with previous RPC–IPAA investigated with MDCT enterography. In the *right* iliac fossa, substenosis (*arrow*) is identified at the transition between the pouch inlet and upstream ileum, with good pouch distension by neutral peroral contrast. The patient was treated conservatively

Fig. 15.13 Functional pouch-anal anastomosis stricture due to mucosal flap, suggested by pouch dilatation without significant mural or perivisceral abnormalities at unenhanced (**a**) and post-contrast (**b**) MRI, already treated with anal dilatation. After negative findings from pouch endoscopy, persistent obstruction investigated with MDCT enterography (**c**, **d**) showed associated malpositioning and torsion of the pouch inlet (*arrows*) causing upstream small bowel dilatation. Surgical treatment including mucosal flap resection was necessary

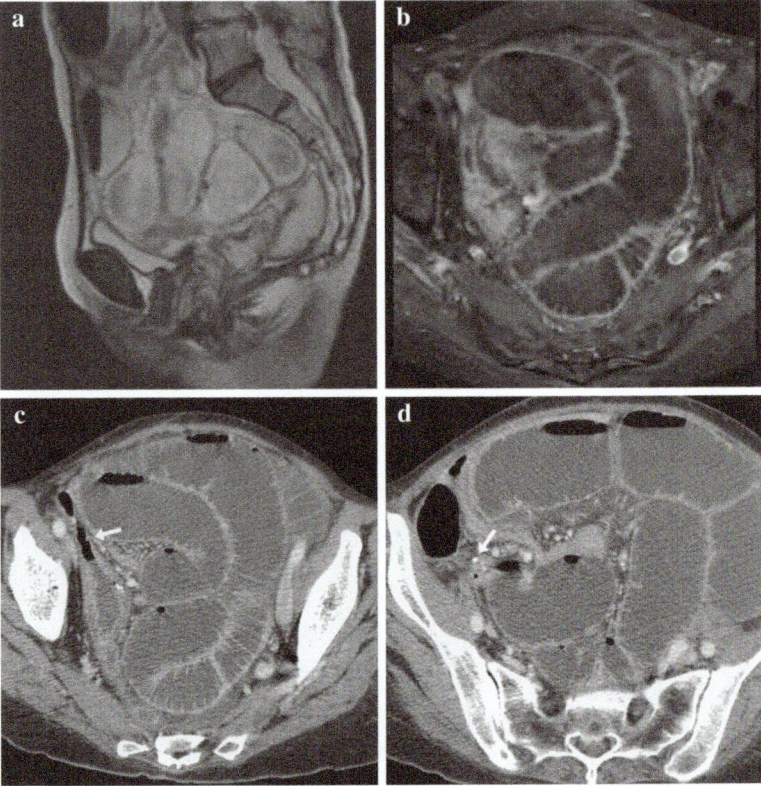

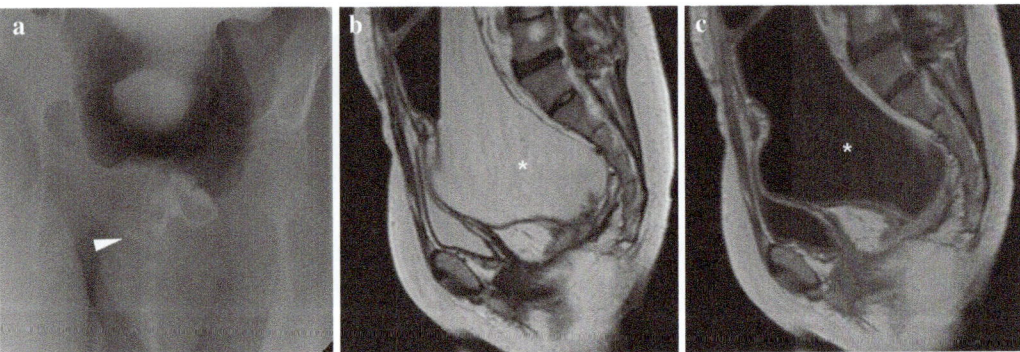

Fig. 15.14 Patient with clinical evidence of anal stenosis and pouch-vaginal fistula. Stenosis of the ileal pouch-anal anastomosis is depicted by double-contrast enema (**a**) with concomitant opacification of anovaginal fistulous tracts (*arrowhead*). MRI shows marked pouch dilatation on sagittal T2-weighted (**b**) and post-contrast T1-weighted (**c**) images [Reprinted with permission from Ref. [11]]

incontinence, pelvic discomfort or crampy abdominal pain, malaise, occasionally with bleeding and low-grade fever. Pouchoscopy and mucosal biopsy should be performed in patients with suspected pouchitis to confirm the diagnosis. Consistent endoscopic findings include an acute, non-specific inflammation with diffuse mucosal oedema, erythema, granularity, friability, spontaneous contact bleeding, loss of vascular pattern, erosions and ulcerations. Histology usually shows acute and chronic inflammation co-existing with microscopic

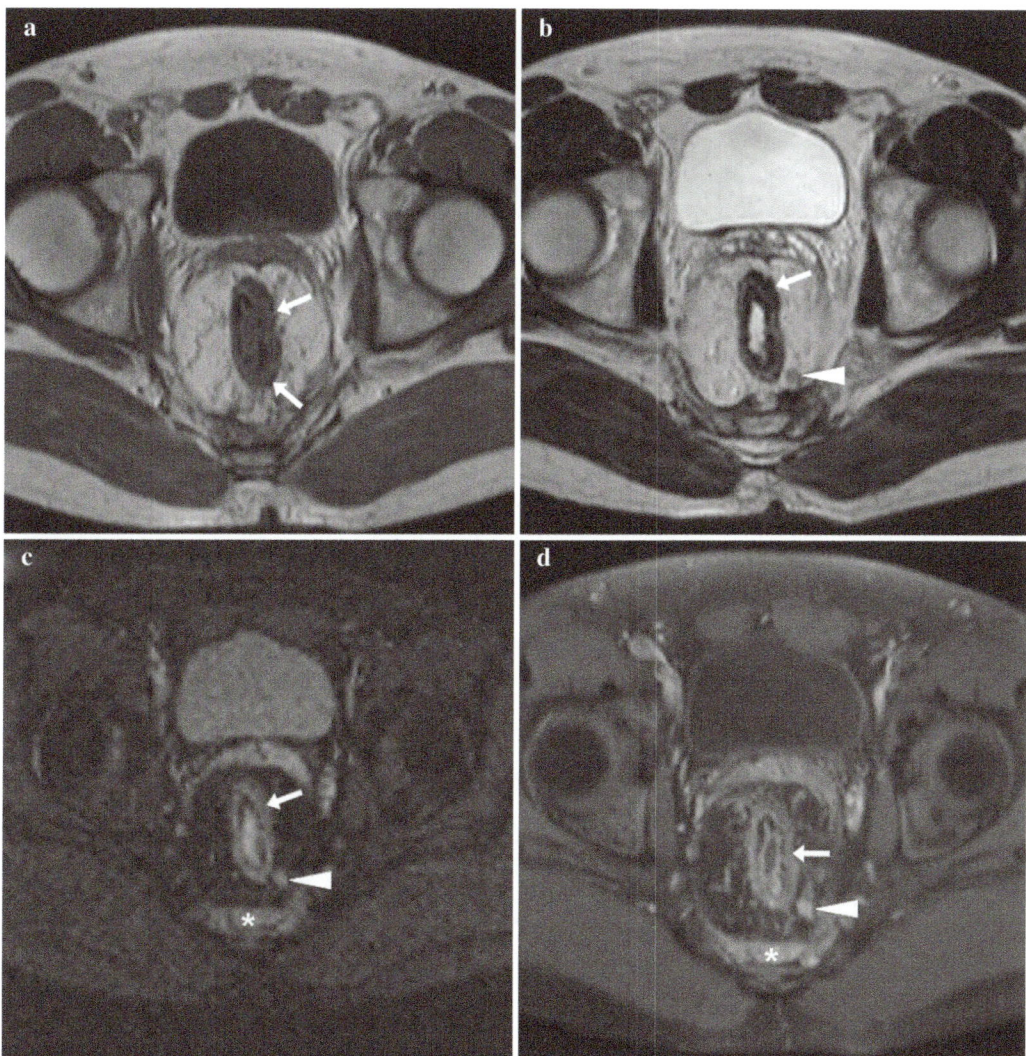

Fig. 15.15 Chronic pouchitis confirmed by endoscopic and bioptic findings. Axial T1- (**a**), T2- (**b**), STIR (**c**) and post-contrast fat-suppressed T1-weighted (**d**) MRI images show circumferential pouch wall thickening (*arrows*) with abnormal signal intensity, discrete enhancement, peripouch fat proliferation and subtle stranding, presence of enhancing lymph nodes (*arrowheads*) [Partly reprinted with permission from Ref. [11]]

ulcers, villous atrophy, crypt distortion or hyperplasia. The severity of complaints may not correlate with the degree of endoscopic and histologic changes [1, 4].

The treatment of pouchitis is empirical, and the majority of patients improve with prolonged courses of antibiotics such as metronidazole and ciprofloxacin, plus other medications including probiotics, infliximab and oral or enema steroids. Unfortunately, pouchitis recurs in more than 50 % of patients [1, 4, 27–29].

In our previously reported experience, contrast-enhanced MRI has proven invaluable for the diagnostic assessment of patients with suspected pouch-related complications, allowing the differentiation of uncomplicated pouchitis from pelvic sepsis. MRI features consistent with pouchitis include pouch wall thickening

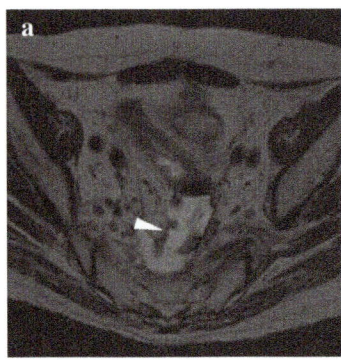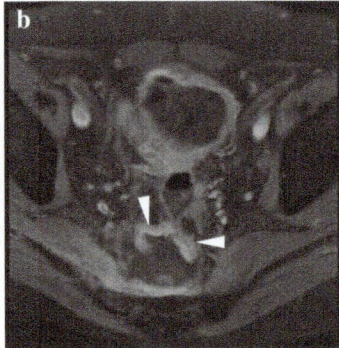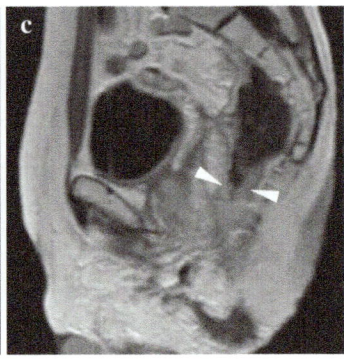

Fig. 15.16 Carcinoma developing in the ileal pouch in a patient with previous restorative proctocolectomy for ulcerative colitis with dysplastic and malignant changes. After endoscopic finding of mucosal irregularities, axial T2- (**a**), post-contrast fat-saturated axial (**b**) and sagittal (**c**) T1-weighted MRI images shows eccentric mural thickening of the ileal pouch (*arrowheads*) with solid signal intensity and positive enhancement. Biopsy confirmed superimposed carcinoma

(>2 mm) and positive contrast enhancement, commonly presence of lymphadenopathies (at least 3 peripouch nodes or one >1 cm), proliferation and inflammatory stranding of the peripouch fat (Fig. 15.15) [11].

Imaging findings of thickening and enhancement of the pouch wall constantly correlate with an erythematous ulcerated mucosa at endoscopy, and with active inflammation and ulceration at histology. Furthermore, a normal MRI has been reported to be a good negative predictor of pouch disease [17].

disease irrespective of IPAA duration, a preoperative, intraoperative or pathologic diagnosis of dysplasia or cancer superimposed of UC, persistent inflammation and/or villous atrophy of the ileal pouch mucosa [3].

Cross-sectional imaging helpfully complements pouch endoscopy, particularly when suspected changes are detected. On MDCT and MRI, the presence of solid-appearing wall thickening with positive contrast enhancement, or the appearance of size and/or mural modifications in the pouch wall should be viewed with suspect, and biopsy should be suggested (Fig. 15.16) [2, 3, 7].

15.4   Pouch Dysplasia and Neoplasia

Surgical treatment of UC with RPC and IPAA dramatically reduces the risk for colonic dysplastic and malignant changes that may sometimes develop in the rectal cuff or in the ileal pouch mucosa. Although the natural history is not well understood, colon carcinoma arising from pouch metaplasia has been exceptionally reported [2, 3, 7].

Since no clear recommendations exist on surveillance of pouches with respect to malignant changes, follow-up of IPAA patients should be individualized and focused on those patients with risk factors such as co-existent primary sclerosing cholangitis, longer duration of UC

References

1. Biancone L, Michetti P, Travis S et al (2008) European evidence-based consensus on the management of ulcerative colitis: special situations. J Crohns Colitis 2:63–92
2. Travis SP, Stange EF, Lemann M et al (2008) European evidence-based consensus on the management of ulcerative colitis: current management. J Crohns Colitis 2:24–62
3. Dignass A, Lindsay JO, Sturm A et al (2012) Second European evidence-based consensus on the diagnosis and management of ulcerative colitis part 2: current management. J Crohns Colitis 6:991–1030
4. Van Assche G, Dignass A, Bokemeyer B et al (2013) Second European evidence-based consensus on the diagnosis and management of ulcerative colitis Part 3: special situations. J Crohns Colitis 7:1–33

5. Hueting WE, Buskens E, van der Tweel I et al (2005) Results and complications after ileal pouch anal anastomosis: a meta-analysis of 43 observational studies comprising 9,317 patients. Dig Surg 22:69–79

6. Hahnloser D, Pemberton JH, Wolff BG et al (2007) Results at up to 20 years after ileal pouch-anal anastomosis for chronic ulcerative colitis. Br J Surg 94:333–340

7. Shen B, Remzi FH, Lavery IC, et al (2008) A proposed classification of ileal pouch disorders and associated complications after restorative proctocolectomy. Clin Gastroenterol Hepatol 6:145-158; quiz 124

8. Alfisher MM, Scholz FJ, Roberts PL, et al (1997) Radiology of ileal pouch-anal anastomosis: normal findings, examination pitfalls, and complications. Radiographics 17:81-98; discussion 98-89

9. Seggerman RE, Chen MY, Waters GS et al (2003) Pictorial essay. radiology of ileal pouch-anal anastomosis surgery. AJR Am J Roentgenol 180:999–1002

10. Crema MD, Richarme D, Azizi L et al (2006) Pouchography, CT, and MRI features of ileal J pouch-anal anastomosis. AJR Am J Roentgenol 187:W594–W603

11. Tonolini M, Campari A, Bianco R (2011) Ileal pouch and related complications: spectrum of imaging findings with emphasis on MRI. Abdom Imaging 36:698–706

12. Mazzeo S, Caramella D, Belcari A et al (2005) Multidetector CT of the small bowel: evaluation after oral hyperhydration with isotonic solution. Radiol Med 109:516–526

13. Lee SS, Kim AY, Yang SK et al (2009) Crohn disease of the small bowel: comparison of CT enterography, MR enterography, and small-bowel follow-through as diagnostic techniques. Radiol 251:751–761

14. Elsayes KM, Al-Hawary MM, Jagdish J et al (2010) CT enterography: principles, trends, and interpretation of findings. Radiogr 30:1955–1970

15. Broder JC, Tkacz JN, Anderson SW et al (2010) Ileal pouch-anal anastomosis surgery: imaging and intervention for post-operative complications. Radiogr 30:221–233

16. Hoeffel C, Arrive L, Mourra N et al (2006) Anatomic and pathologic findings at external phased-array pelvic MR imaging after surgery for anorectal disease. Radiogr 26:1391–1407

17. Nadgir RN, Soto JA, Dendrinos K et al (2006) MRI of complicated pouchitis. AJR Am J Roentgenol 187:W386–W391

18. Tang L, Cai H, Moore L et al (2010) Evaluation of endoscopic and imaging modalities in the diagnosis of structural disorders of the ileal pouch. Inflamm Bowel Dis 16:1526–1531

19. Zissin R, Hertz M, Paran H et al (2004) Small bowel obstruction secondary to Crohn disease: CT findings. Abdom Imaging 29:320–325

20. Silva AC, Pimenta M, Guimaraes LS (2009) Small bowel obstruction: what to look for. Radiogr 29:423–439

21. Beliard A, Prudhomme M (2010) Ileal reservoir with ileo-anal anastomosis: long-term complications. J Visc Surg 147:e137–e144

22. Fazio VW, Ziv Y, Church JM et al (1995) Ileal pouch-anal anastomoses complications and function in 1005 patients. Ann Surg 222:120–127

23. Nahon S, Cadranel JF, Chazouilleres O et al (2009) Liver and inflammatory bowel disease. Gastroenterol Clin Biol 33:370–381

24. Remzi FH, Fazio VW, Oncel M, et al (2002) Portal vein thrombi after restorative proctocolectomy. Surgery 132:655-661; discussion 661-652

25. Ball CG, MacLean AR, Buie WD et al (2007) Portal vein thrombi after ileal pouch-anal anastomosis: its incidence and association with pouchitis. Surg Today 37:552–557

26. Simchuk EJ, Thirlby RC (2000) Risk factors and true incidence of pouchitis in patients after ileal pouch-anal anastomoses. World J Surg 24:851–856

27. Pardi DS, Sandborn WJ (2006) Systematic review: the management of pouchitis. Aliment Pharmacol Ther 23:1087–1096

28. Akerlund JE, Lofberg R (2004) Pouchitis. Curr Opin Gastroenterol 20:341–344

29. Cheifetz A, Itzkowitz S (2004) The diagnosis and treatment of pouchitis in inflammatory bowel disease. J Clin Gastroenterol 38:S44–S50

Index

GPSR Compliance

*The European Union's (EU) General Product Safety Regulation (GPSR)
is a set of rules that requires consumer products to be safe and our
obligations to ensure this.*

*If you have any concerns about our products, you can contact us on
ProductSafety@springernature.com*

In case Publisher is established outside the EU, the EU authorized
representative is:

Springer Nature Customer Service Center GmbH
Europaplatz 3
69115 Heidelberg, Germany

Batoh number: 09635705

Printed by Printforce, the Netherlands